Breastfeeding: A Mother's Gift

Pamela K. Wiggins, IBCLC

L. A. Publishing Company, Franklin, Virginia

Breastfeeding: A Mother's Gift

by Pamela K. Wiggins, IBCLC

L. A. Publishing Company
30149 Smiths Ferry Road
P. O. Box 773
Franklin, Virginia 23851
(757) 562-2223

LAP © Copyright 1998

ISBN # 0-9623529-6-9
Library of Congress Catalog Number: 97-92730

Publisher's Cataloging-in-Publication
(Provided by Quality Books, Inc.)

Wiggins, Pamela.
    Breastfeeding: a mother's gift/Pamela K. Wiggins.--
Rev. 2nd ed.
    p.cm.
    Includes bibliographical references and index.
    ISBN: 0-9623529-6-9

    1. Breast feeding   I. Title.
    RJ216.W65   1998   649'.33
                        QBI97-41379

Dedication

This book is dedicated to my husband and my children, who are the lights of my life.

And to all women, everywhere, who have made the right choice: to breastfeed.

Cover Photo: Laura Solomon
Art Director: Joanna Wiggins

Photo credits:

Laura Soloman, pp. 24,142
Nifty Nurser, p.95
Over the Shoulder Baby Holder, p.86
Kay Hoover, pp. 58,93,98,119
(Information about these photos and breastfeeding slide sets may be obtained from Kay Hoover, 613 Yale Ave., Morton PA 19070)

- **NOTE:** The author realizes that babies come in both sexes, but for the sake of simplicity, will refer to the baby as "he" throughout this booklet. She apologizes to all baby girls.

ACKNOWLEDGEMENTS

I couldn't possibly go to press without mentioning the people who have helped me put this book together.

My sincere thanks to:

Joanna - my daughter, a second-generation breastfeeding advocate, who helped with editorial matters and art direction. Her help was invaluable.

Katherine Dettwyler, the distinguished anthropologist, who wrote the foreword.

Tom Hale, the famous author-professor, who wrote the section on "Using Medications in the Breastfeeding Mother."

Chanita Stillerman-Evans, a wonderful and knowledgeable editor, who not only edited the book, but provided many ideas and suggestions, some of which I have used in their entirety.

Laura, my best friend and cover model, and to her little sons, Blayne and Harrison (and my godsons), who posed so nicely.

My models, Lorij, Carlette, Debbie, Judith, Cherie, Sally, Ruth, Karen, Sherie, and their sweet babies, and to little Janice, too.

Kay Hoover who provided photographs as noted.

I couldn't have done it without any of you!

TABLE OF CONTENTS

Foreword

Katherine A. Dettwyler, Ph.D.

This is a book about breastfeeding, but it's also a book about choice. This is a book about why women should choose to breastfeed their babies, but it's also a book about how to be successful at it. This is a book about possible problems one might encounter with breastfeeding, but it's also a book about how to deal with those problems. You might find yourself asking, why is a book like this necessary? Isn't breastfeeding natural?

Humans are mammals, members of the Class Mammalia, along with cats, rabbits, zebras, and chimpanzees. For some mammals, nurturing their young with their mammary glands is instinctual—they don't have to think about it, they don't have to learn how to do it, and they don't have to "choose" this method of infant care. For the primates, however, many activities that are purely instinctual in other animals have a large learned component. This is especially true for our closest relatives, the great apes—chimpanzees, gorillas, and orangutans. Young female chimpanzees learn how to be good mothers by observing their own mothers and aunts and cousins rearing their young. When their time comes to nurture their own offspring, they know what to do. Likewise, women who grow up in breastfeeding cultures learn all about how breastfeeding works by observing their relatives, friends, and neighbors care for their children at the breast. They can ask questions and participate in discussions of how to overcome common difficulties. Everyone nurses their children, and assumes that everyone else will too - it's just how children are fed and cared for - no one has to "choose" to breastfeed.

I was very fortunate to have been breastfed, even though, as a Baby-Boomer, I was born at a time when breastfeeding was not the norm. I never gave it much thought growing up, but was fortunate again to have a good friend who was breastfeeding her son when I became pregnant with my first child. She took me to La Leche League meetings, and talked at great length about how important and satisfying breastfeeding was for both mother and child. And so for me, there really was no choice to be made either - of course I would do what was natural and normal and best for my child. When my daughter was 15 months old, I left the U.S. to go to the West African country of Mali, to do research on infant and child feeding, and for two years I lived enmeshed in a breastfeeding culture. In Mali in the early 1980s, all women breastfed their children, on cue, including at night, in every possible circumstance. I saw women breastfeeding at home, in the fields, in the markets, on public transportation - everywhere there were women there were women breastfeeding children. I learned about Malian beliefs that a mother becomes related to her children by breastfeeding them, and I learned that breastfeeding is easy when everyone around you supports it.

When I returned to the United States, I became more aware of the many cultural forces that make it difficult for many women to choose to breastfeed in the U. S. These include the sexualization of the breasts in U. S. culture, the lack of training available to health care providers that would allow them to help mothers breastfeed, and the power of the infant formula companies to convince women that breastfeeding really doesn't matter, and that infant formula is just as good.

But breastfeeding does matter. There's an old saying: "If you don't know your options, you don't have any." This book, with its clear and engaging style, provides readers with the information they need to have a real option to choose breastfeeding as the best way to nurture their children.

Katherine A. Dettwyler is the co-editor of <u>Breastfeeding: Biocultural Perspectives</u> *(1995, Aldine De Gruyter, New York) and author of* <u>Dancing Skeletons</u>, *winner of the 1995 Margaret Mead Award for the best interpretation of anthropological research for a lay audience. (1995, Waveland Press, Inc. Prospect Heights, IL)*

The Author's Story

It wasn't popular to breastfeed in 1973. In fact, in the small Virginia town where I lived, I didn't personally know *any* women who had nursed their babies. And it had never crossed MY mind until my husband and I took an expectant parents' class at the local community college.

The class, taught by two Red Cross nurses, was made up of about 10 couples, all about as ignorant of parenting as we were. We learned the basics: how to bathe a baby, change diapers, and how to mix formula. Both nurses had actually breastfed their children for a while, and they mentioned it as a feeding option. They even said it was "better" than formula feeding. But no instruction was given, and when they asked if anyone planned to breastfeed, not a single hand went up. However, the seed was planted. And somehow I just *knew* that breastfeeding was the right thing to do. Afterwards my husband and I discussed it a little, and he, being a good farm boy, commented that he liked the idea, and hoped I would try it. (He knew all about colostrum and how calves couldn't survive without it.) I can't remember discussing it again, or even reading anything about it before my son was born.

Joe was born on the day of Nixon's inauguration. The birth did not go as planned, and after 24 hours of hard labor, I had a Cesarean section. Back then, Cesareans were a big deal. (And they still are, in my opinion.) I had private duty nurses who sat with me around the clock for 2 days, and visiting was limited to the immediate family. I got to see my son on the morning of the second day.

Thankfully, my little son knew more about breastfeeding than I did. He latched right on, and nursed for 5 minutes on each side, just as the nurse had instructed. She was very disappointed that I insisted on nursing, because, after all, I had just had major surgery, and nursing would "make things

15

worse."

The breastfeeding protocol in the hospital was that they would bring my baby to me every four hours, except during the night, when they would let me get my rest! If my baby got hungry before the four hours, or during the night, they would give him either water or formula. Oh, how little I knew, and how obedient and docile I was then.

I was instructed to wash my nipples with alcohol-soaked cotton balls and to rinse with sterile water. To this day, I can hear those two nursery nurses plodding down the corridor - one carrying my baby and the other carrying a stainless steel tray that held the jingling jars of alcohol and sterile water.

By the third day, I was heavily engorged and sore, Joe was jaundiced, and post-partum depression was settling in fast. But I hung in there, nursing every four hours on the dot.

And after 7 long days, they finally let me go home - but without my baby! He had to stay another 3 days, under the phototherapy lights, until his bilirubin count went down to the magic number, "8." I was allowed to visit and breastfeed my baby twice a day, and because of the sore nipples, advised to wear hard rubber nipple shields. At home, I used a bicycle horn pump to relieve engorgement, and the milk was discarded. No one ever told me I could save it.

Finally, I located an old navy-blue copy of La Leche League's *Womanly Art of Breastfeeding*. I learned much from that book. I learned about demand feeding and how long to nurse. And I learned about LLL meetings and how to contact a leader. And finally, after many long distance phone calls, I located one. When Joe was 3 months old, I went to my first LLL meeting. It was 70 miles away.

The rest, as they say, is history! I fell in love with my baby and with breastfeeding. By the time my daughter came along, I had become an LLL Leader, and I knew what I was doing. And by the time my second son came along, I knew that mothering and lactation consulting would be my life's work. I became a board certified lactation consultant in 1985, and wrote *Why Should I Nurse My Baby?* three years later. The success of that little book enabled me to do what I like doing best - staying at home with my children.

Each of my children was nurtured at my breasts for a long, long time, and received the very best I had to give. As I look back, I'm glad I gave my children the best possible start. They have all turned out to be responsible young adults who are confident, well-behaved, and unafraid to try new things.

I credit a relaxed style of parenting, faith in the Lord, and breastfeeding for the successes my husband and I have had in our family.

When a child is unconditionally loved, taught correct principles, and fed at the breast, he will grow up more self-reliant and confident. And although breastfeeding (*or* unconditionally loving a child) is not always easy, **it is worth it**. I know, without a doubt, that I made the right choice when I decided to breastfeed my children.

Introduction

Breastfeeding is the very best gift you can give your child. It will provide him with health and emotional benefits that will last the rest of his life.

Indeed, your decision about whether to breastfeed or bottle-feed is one of the most important decisions you will ever have to make. And this book, by thoroughly discussing the many benefits, and by implying the risks of feeding artificial baby milk, is designed to help you make the right decision.

Breastfeeding is the best possible way of nourishing your infant and ensuring optimal health. It is not only better than artificial feeding, but is actually the "normal" way of infant feeding. According to the World Health Organization, choices in infant feeding are, first, breastfeeding (*your* baby suckling at *your* breast); second, feeding your baby your own milk from a bottle or via other mechanism; third, feeding human breast milk from a donor mother; and fourth, giving your baby formula. Formula comes in FOURTH! Babies who don't breastfeed, and who are not fed human breastmilk, may survive, and even do well. However, research shows that this puts most babies at a disadvantage physically, psychologically, and mentally.

Mother's milk has many unique attributes that formula does not have. It actually has *live* cells that provide important immunities and these, along with the best possible nutrients, will help keep your baby healthy and well. Researchers who study human breastmilk are finding out more every day about this "liquid gold." They are now rediscovering what Mother Nature has known all along - that breastmilk is far superior to any other infant food, and that it is much more than just food.

The emotional benefit of breastfeeding is another gift you can give your child. Throughout the nursing relationship, he will receive love and security at your breast, and will learn to trust others. By giving of yourself through nursing, your baby's emotional needs will be met, and he will likely grow up to be a secure, well-adjusted adult.

The mental benefits of breastfeeding are only now being discovered, but several reliable studies indicate that the cognitive development and Intelligence Quotients of breastfed children are much more advanced.

Mothers have breastfed their babies since the beginning of humankind. However, when mothers died or became sick alternatives had to be found. If another woman's milk wasn't available, then animal milk or a gruel-like substance, made from grains, was used. Eventually scientists began to create breastmilk substitutes for these special circumstances. It has only been in the last sixty or so years that large companies have aggressively promoted breastmilk substitutes for *all* mothers and babies.

In the 1950s, when pregnancy, birth, and feeding methods became more "medicalized," the use of breastmilk substitutes became normal. As a result, formula companies had an increasingly lucrative market in providing manufactured baby milk to mothers who didn't want to breastfeed.

Today these very same formula companies are very aggressive in their marketing techniques. They influence many to believe that formula is "just as good" as mother's milk. From the moment they find out you're pregnant (and somehow, they know) to the moment you leave the hospital, with their free formula samples in hand, you are being influenced to feed your baby an inferior food.

Due to the pervasiveness of formula, and the general ignorance of the **value** of human milk, breastfeeding "went out of style" in the United States (and other industrialized countries) for a long, long time, and most mothers today have not grown up in a world where women routinely breastfeed.

And for that reason and many others, breastfeeding doesn't always seem like the normal way of infant feeding. And it doesn't always come naturally to the mother. Sometimes it must be taught.

That is why *Breastfeeding: A Mother's Gift* was written. The long list of benefits in chapter one will convince you (or confirm what you've heard) of the value of breastfeeding, and the subsequent chapters will teach you how to do it successfully. It will help you gain the confidence you need to give your baby that wonderful gift: your milk. Please refer to this book after your baby is born.

Your baby has the **right** to get the very best from you. Why not give him the most precious gifts of all? Love, nourishment, and security from your breast. **You will both benefit from it!**

Chapter One

The Benefits of Breastfeeding

I wouldn't take anything for the experience of breastfeeding my children. They are happy and healthy. What more could a mother ask? I have never regretted nursing my babies.

Linda

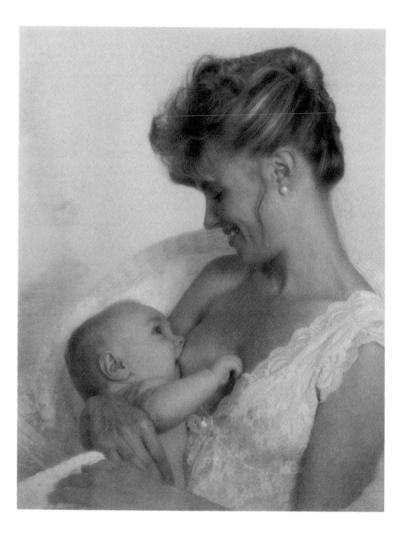

The Benefits
Of Breastfeeding

Mothers have many reasons for nursing their babies. Some just see it as the normal way of feeding infants, and don't really think much about the physical and emotional benefits. Others just know in their hearts it is the right thing to do. Still others have heard of the advantages, and they want to give the best to their children.

Then, there are those who have probably heard some of the benefits, and are seriously considering breastfeeding, but are not quite convinced it is really better.

Whether you have already decided, or if you are still in the "thinking" stage, read this chapter carefully. It lists the many benefits, and is referenced for further investigation. It should help convince you that breastfeeding is important to the physical, mental and emotional health of your child, and that it is the very best thing you can do for yourself, your baby and the earth.

Breastfeeding is best for your BABY.

•   Human breastmilk is the perfect food for your baby. It has all the right ingredients in just the right amounts. It contains the proper amounts of fatty acids, lactose, water and amino acids for optimal growth, digestion and brain development. Your body knows *exactly* what your baby needs nutritionally, and provides it through your own milk. Your body provided for your baby in utero, and will continue to do so during lactation. All milk that comes from animals is "species-specific." Just as cow milk is for calves, cat milk is for kittens, and so on, human milk is for human babies. We all belong to the class **mammalia** which means we feed our young milk from our mammary glands. Did you know that humans are the only species that ever feeds its young the milk from another species?

• Breastfeeding will help you and you baby "bond" with one another. There will be a special closeness between you that will last a long time. Prolactin, a hormone released when the baby suckles, will help you to have those special "mothering" feelings. It is also a natural tranquilizer, and will help you feel relaxed and peaceful while nursing. Finally, prolactin triggers a fierce protective mechanism in mothers. Because of both the bonding and the protective responses triggered, some experts think breastfeeding may help reduce future child abuse. [1]

• Mother's milk is easily digested. Artificial baby milk (formula) is usually made from cow's milk, and the large amounts of protein (suitable for growing calves) make it hard for human babies to digest. The proteins found in human milk are all put to use by the baby, whereas only about half of the proteins found in formulas are digested.

• Breastfed infants seldom get diarrhea, but when they do, it is usually a mild case and easily treated. [2,3] They are much less likely to develop complications from it. Breastmilk is not contaminated with germs that might cause diarrhea. One study found that bottle-fed babies are fourteen times more likely to die from diarrhea than exclusively breastfed infants.[4]

• Breastfed babies have fewer allergies than artificially fed babies. This is especially important if your family has a history of allergies. Many babies are allergic to cow's milk formulas. Some babies are even allergic to soy formulas. Breastfeeding protects against other allergies, such as atopic eczema, food allergies, and respiratory allergies.[5,6]

• The antibodies in breastmilk will provide immunities that will help protect your baby from common ailments like colds, flu, sore throats, ear infections, (7,8) and more serious illnesses like childhood lymphomas and cancers, (9,10) juvenile diabetes, (11,12) Crohns disease, (13) and ulcerative colitis.(14) These antibodies provide protection for many months. In fact, even after your baby is eating solids and not nursing as often, he will still be getting protective antibodies. As long as your baby is getting your milk, he is getting "preventive medicine."

• Studies suggest that breastfeeding reduces the risk of SIDS (Sudden Infant Death Syndrome). In fact, one important study found that for each month of exclusive breastfeeding, the risk of SIDS is reduced by half, when compared to formula-fed infants.(15, 16) Some factors at work in these findings are: breastfeeding reduces the danger of botulism poisoning and the danger of breathing problems associated with respiratory infections. It reduces the incidence of breathing problems associated with slower brain development, which is found in formula-fed infants. And breastfed babies have lighter sleep cycles, which reduces the risk of apnea and sleep arousal problems.

• Breastfed babies have stronger and straighter teeth which means they probably won't need braces.(17) The tongue action is unique in breastfeeding infants and affects the way teeth grow in. The length of time a child is breastfed also affects the outcome - the longer the child is breastfed, the less likely his or her teeth will grow in crooked or crowded. Most breastfed children have fewer dental caries, too.(18)

• Breastfed babies are easily comforted at the breast, especially when they are sick or hurt. Mothers appreciate this special way they can comfort their babies when they are in pain or ill or just cross. Comforting your baby at your breast (even when he is not hungry) will help your baby feel secure and loved. Most breastfed babies don't cry as much as bottle babies, because they are so easily comforted at the mother's breast. Believe it or not, there are many breastfed babies who seldom cry at all. Their mothers are so "tuned in" to their signals, that they can comfort them before they even start crying.

• Because of the special way they suckle, breastfed babies have fewer speech problems than bottle-fed babies. Their tongues and jaw muscles are exercised in just the right way.[19]

• Breastfed babies are not likely to be overweight. Since they control how much they take (demand feeding) they don't overfeed. They get exactly the right amount of calories for their needs. And if a baby does happen to gain a few extra pounds during the early months, he will probably lose it when he becomes more active. Bottle-fed babies are often overfed, and they frequently gain too much. This extra weight is often carried into childhood and adolescence and even into adulthood.

• Studies have found that breastfed babies have higher IQs than formula-fed babies. There are factors in human breast milk that enhance brain development and improve cognitive development.[20-22] One study found that the average IQ of 7 and 8 year olds, who had been breastfed, was 10 points higher than their bottle-fed counterparts.[23] This study is important because it studied pre-term infants that had been tube-fed human milk while hospitalized, so it was clearly something in the milk itself, not the act of breastfeeding. It also included adjustments for differences between groups and the mother's educational and social class.

• Breastfeeding gives your baby the best emotional start. Not only does a child receive the best nutritional start, but many of his emotional needs are met at the breast. A child who receives love and security at his mother's breast grows up with self-confidence and trust. The emotional advantages of breastfeeding are very important.

• Breastmilk even affects vaccinations. Children who are breastfed show a better antibody response to vaccines than formula-fed children.(24)

Breastfeeding is best for YOU.

• Breastmilk is always available and at the right temperature. It is nature's convenience food! You will be able to feed your baby when he is hungry - any time and any place. When you go places, you don't have to pack up bottles, sterilizing equipment, and formula. And you will always have food for your baby, even in a disaster. Did you ever wonder how bottle-fed babies are fed during a hurricane or flood or some other natural disaster? Not only might the stores be closed, but the water used to mix powdered formula might be contaminated.

• Nighttime feedings are much easier when you breastfeed. Just tuck baby in bed with you, and you can both go back to sleep. You will not have to trudge to the kitchen and warm up a bottle in the middle of the night, while baby is screaming. Some parents find this advantage to be the best one of all. And many parents find sleeping with their babies nearby or in bed with them to be the ideal situation. In fact, in most cultures around the world, this is the normal thing to do. Your baby needs *you* more than a room of his own.

•   It is much more economical to breastfeed than to bottle feed. Breastmilk is free. You don't have to buy expensive formula, sterilizing kits, bottles, nipples and warmers. The average formula costs about $1000 per year. Special formulas, for babies with allergies, cost MUCH more. Since breastfed babies are not sick as often, there are fewer doctor bills to pay. A recent study showed that breastfed babies are much less likely to be admitted to a hospital during the first year.(25) Breastfeeding could save you (or your insurance company) huge amounts of money.

•   Your breastfed baby will always know YOU are his mother. Working mothers often worry that the baby will become too attached to the caregiver. And occasionally, that happens. But even if you are only nursing part-time, you will still be the center of your child's life.

•   When you breastfeed, your body will get back to its pre-pregnancy state faster. As the baby suckles, a hormone (oxytocin) is released which causes the uterus to contract. It helps prevent excessive bleeding and helps return the uterus to its non-pregnant size.

•   Breastfeeding will help you lose the weight you put on during pregnancy. As long as you don't over-eat, you should be able to gradually shed those extra pounds and keep them off.

•   Recent studies suggest that breastfeeding helps prevent some cancers in the mother. The risk of breast cancer is higher in women who bottle-feed their children, and is also higher in women who were not breastfed as children.(26-28) Thus, breastfeeding your daughters is a way to provide a special gift to them - extra protection against breast cancer. Recent studies also suggest that breastfeeding reduces the risk of uterine, (29) ovarian (30-32) and endometrial cancers.(33) It is thought that the suppression of certain hormones during lactation is a factor in these risks.

• Breastfeeding gives you a sense of self worth and a feeling you have contributed to society. It empowers you because you can see the value of what you are doing. It encourages self-reliance because you gain confidence in yourself as you meet the needs of your baby. It "confirms a woman's power to control her own body, and challenges the male-dominated medical model, and business interests that promote bottle feeding." (World Alliance for Breastfeeding Action)

• Two little known advantages to women are that breast-feeding may bring about a decrease in insulin requirements in diabetic women (34) and it may also decrease the risk of osteoporosis.(35)

• You probably won't have a menstrual period as long as you are exclusively breastfeeding. And you *probably* won't ovulate until you have your first period. Exclusive breastfeed-ing (no bottles or pacifiers) offers **some** protection from pregnancy for the first few months. It is nature's way of spacing babies. (36)

• Breastfed babies smell good. Because breastmilk is all natural, their breath is pleasant and their stools don't smell bad. And most breastfed babies don't spit up. If they do, it is usually because they have just had a bit too much. It won't smell sour or stain clothes.

Breastfeeding is also best for the EARTH.

• Breastfeeding saves our natural resources and does not pollute. Formula-feeding, on the other hand, contributes to massive amounts of solid waste (bottles, cans, etc.) and the production of formula requires excessive amounts of energy, water, plastic, paper and tin. The manufacturing of baby bottles also requires energy, glass, plastic, and rubber. And the feeding of cows (cow's milk being the main ingredient in most formulas) takes valuable land, water, and food, and pollutes water and air.

Breastfeeding does not cost money, cause waste or use valuable natural resources. It is the most "politically correct" way of feeding infants.

The list of advantages here is important, but is by no means complete. Every day, researchers are learning more about the wonders of mother's milk. Please read the references if you want to learn more about some of the recent research relating to infant feeding.

Breastfeeding is the very best gift you can give - to **yourself** and **your baby** and the **earth**!

References

(1) Acheson, L., Family Violence and Breastfeeding. *Archives Family Medicine*, 1995; vol. 4, 650-52.

(2) Feachem, R. G. and Koblinsky, M. A. Interventions for the Control of Diarrhoeal Diseases Among Children. Promotion of Breastfeeding. *Bulletin of the World Health Organization*, 1984; 62.

(3) Huffman, S. et al. Role of Breastfeeding in the Prevention and Treatment of Diarrhoea. *Journal of Diarrhoeal Disease, 1990*; 8:68-81.

(4) Victora, C., et al. Infant Feedings and Deaths Due to Diarrhea: A Case-Controlled Study. *American Journal of Epidemiology*, 1989; 129.

(5) Saarinen, U. M. et al., Breastfeeding as Prophylaxis Against Atopic Disease: Prospective Follow-up Study Until 17 Years Old. *Lancet*, 1995; 1065-69.

(6) Merrett, T. G., et al. Infant Feeding and Allergy: Twelve Month Prospective Study of 500 Babies Born in Allergic Families. *American Allergy*, 1988; 13-20.

(7) Dewey, K. G. et al. Differences in Morbidity Between Breastfed and Formula Fed Infants. *Journal of Pediatrics*, 1995; 1: 696-702.

(8) Howie, P.W., et al. Protective Effect of Breastfeeding Against Infection. *British Medical Journal,1990*; 300:11-16.

(9) Davis, M. et al. Infant Feeding and Childhood Lymphomas. *Lancet*, 1988; 2:365-68.

(10) Schwartzbaum, J. et al. An Exploratory Study of Environmental and Medical Factors Potentially Related to Childhood Cancer. *Medical Pediatrics Oncology*, 1992; 115-21.

(11) Borch-Johnson, K., et al., Relation Between Breastfeeding and Incidence of Insulin Dependent Diabetes Mellitus. *Lancet*, 1984; 2(8411).

(12) Mayer E. J., et al. Reduced Risk of Insulin Dependent Diabetes Mellitus Among Breastfed Children. *Diabetes*, 1988; 37:1625-32.

(13) Koletzko S., et al. Role of Infant Feeding Practices in Development of Chrohn's Disease in Childhood. *British Medical Journal*, 1989; 298:1616-18.

(14) Whorwell, P. H., et al. Bottlefeeding, Early Gastroenteritis and Inflammatory Bowel Disease. *British Medical Journal*, 1979; 1:382.

15) Fredrickson, D. D., et al. Relationship Between Sudden Infant Death Syndrome and Breastfeeding Intensity and Duration. *American Journal of Diseases in Children*, 1993; 147:460.

(16)Ford RPK et al. Breastfeeding and the Risk of Sudden Infant Death Syndrome. *International Journal of Epidemiology* 1993, 22(5):885-890.

(17) Labbok, M. H., Does Breast Feeding Protect Against Malocclusion. *American Journal of Preventive Medicine,* 1987; 3:227-232.

(18) Lucas A., Cole T.J.: Is Breast Feeding a Likely Cause of Dental Caries in young Children? *Journal of American Dental Association,* 1979; 98:21-23.

(19) Broad, Frances E., The Effects of Infant Feeding on Speech Quality. *New Zealand Medical Journal,* 1976; 76:28-31.

(20) Morrow-Tlucak, M. Breast Feeding and Cognitive Development During the First Two Years of Life. *Social Sciences Medicine,1988;* 26: 635-639.

(21) Rogan, W. J. and Gladen, B.C., Breastfeeding and Cognitive Development. *Early Human Development,* 1993; 31:181-193.

(22) Horwood, J. L. and Gergusson, D. M., Breastfeeding and Later Cognitive and Academic Outcomes. *Pediatrics,* 1998; 101:9-14.

(23) Lucas, A. , Breast Milk and Subsequent Intelligence Quotient in Children Born Preterm. *Lancet,* 1992; 339:261-62.

(24) Hahn-Zoric M, et al. Antibody Responses to Parenteral and Oral Vaccines are Impaired by Conventional and Low Protein Formulas as Compared to Breastfeeding. *Acta Paediatrics Scandinavica,* 1990; 79:1137-1142.

(25) Fallat ME. Et al. Breastfeeding Reduces Incidence of Hospital Admissions for Infections in Infants. *Pediatrics,* 1980; 65:1121-24.

(26) Kelsey, K. and E.John. Lactation and the Risk of Breast Cancer. *New England Journal of Medicine,* 1994; 330(2):136-37.

(27) Newcomb, O. et al. Lactation and Reduced Risk of Premenopausal Breast Cancer. *New England Journal of Medicine,* 1994: 330(2)81-87.

(28) Freudheim, J., Exposure to Breast Milk in Infancy and the Risk of Breast Cancer. *Epidemiology*, 1994:5:324-31.

(29) Brock, K. E., Sexual, Reproductive and Contraceptive Risk Factors for Carcinoma-inSitu of the Uterine Cervix in Sydney. *Medical Journal of Australia*, 1989.

(30) Schneider, A. P., Risk Factor for Ovarian Cancer. *New England Journal of Medicine*, 1987; 317: 508-09.

(31) Gwinn M.L., Lee N.C., Rhodes, et al., Pregnancy, Breast Feeding, and Oral Contraceptives and the Risk of Epithelial Ovarian Cancer. *Journal of Clinical Epidemiology* 1990;43:559-68.

(32) Rosenblatt K.A., Thomas D.B., Lactation and the Risk of Epithelial Ovarian Cancer. The WHO Collaborative Study of Neoplasia and Steroid Contraceptives. *International Journal of Epidemiology* 1993; 22:192-7

(33) Rosenblatt K.A., Thomas D.B., Prolonged Lactation and Endometrial Cancer. The WHO Collaborative Study of Neoplasia and Steroid Contraceptives. *International Journal of Epidemiology*, 1995; 24(3):499-503.

(34) Davies, H. A., Insulin Requirements of Diabetic Women Who Breast Feed. *British Medical Journal*, 1989; 209:1357-58.

(35) Blaauw, R., et al., Risk Factors for Development of Osteoporosis in South African Population. *South African Medical Journal*, 1994; 84:328-32.

(36) Thapa, S., Breastfeeding, Child Spacing and Their Effects of Child Survival. *Nature*, 1988; 335:679-82.

Note: Many of these references (and more) are reviewed in: Cunningham, Allan S., "Breastfeeding: Adaptive Behavior for Child Health and Longevity," <u>Breastfeeding: Biocultural Perspectives</u>, 1995; pp. 243-264.

Chapter Two

Preparing to Breastfeed

---

*As soon as I found out I was pregnant,
I started reading everything I could get my
hands on about breastfeeding. I am glad
I did, because everywhere I turned, other
people were telling me stories about how
hard nursing was for them. Knowing
the facts helped me to counter their
negative comments.*

Betty

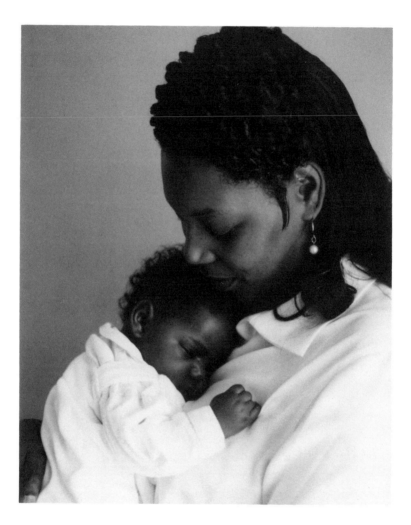

Preparation For Breastfeeding

Preparation for breastfeeding is not physical; it's mental. It consists of learning all you can about breastfeeding before your baby arrives. By reading this book, you are "preparing." There are many other good breastfeeding books and videos available in bookstores, local libraries or La Leche League libraries.

Talk to other mothers who have **successfully** breastfed. If you find yourself listening to a woman who had problems, and who gave up after a few attempts, don't be discouraged. She may not have been as informed or motivated as you will be, or perhaps she just didn't know where to turn for help.

Attend a La Leche League meeting. It is a good place to start meeting breastfeeding moms. There you will find mothers actually nursing their babies - something you may not have seen before. These mothers will gladly help answer your questions, and relate their own reasons for breastfeeding. La Leche League groups have a lending library with lots of good breastfeeding and parenting books.

It is also a good idea to take a breastfeeding class before the baby arrives. Many hospitals and birthing centers now offer breastfeeding classes, and some even make it part of childbirth classes.

Your partner should learn about breastfeeding, too. (At the very least, encourage him to read the first chapter of this book so that he will learn all the advantages.) Having a supportive partner who understands the *value* of breastfeeding is very important.

The following will cover the only physical problem you should be concerned about while still pregnant.

Inverted and Flat Nipples

Be sure and tell your doctor or midwife that you plan to breastfeed, and have him (or her) examine your nipples to see if they are flat or inverted.

The examination is simple. You can even do it yourself. Gently pinch the base of each nipple. **Inverted** nipples go in when they are pinched, and normal nipples stick out. **Flat** nipples stick out, but look somewhat flat. It is fairly common to have flat nipples, but it is extremely rare to have completely inverted nipples. But even if you do, you can almost always overcome this problem. You may need to get **breast shells**.

Breast shells are little plastic devices that are worn in your bra during the last months of pregnancy to help bring out inverted nipples. They work by putting pressure around the base of the nipple, which pushes the nipple out. If they are worn several hours a day in the last trimester, they should bring the nipple out before the baby arrives. But, even if you don't use them until after the baby comes, they will still work. Just wear them between feedings. It may take a few weeks for the nipple to start improving. You can buy breast shells at most maternity stores, LLL Leaders, or from a lactation consultant. See chapter 6 for more about breast shells.

If you have flat or *slightly* inverted nipples, you may be able to gently pull them out with your fingers (far enough out for the baby to latch on to). And some mothers have been able to get them to stand out by putting a cold cloth on them. Be patient and keep trying. The baby's suckling should eventually draw the nipple out.

Some mothers have used **nipple shields** with inverted nipples. Although they may work, they may also be a source of other problems. They can be a factor in decreasing your milk supply, and babies can become "hooked" on them. The hazards of nipple shields are discussed further in chapter 6.

Nipple Preparation

Speaking of nipples, you may have heard that you have to"toughen" up your nipples before the baby comes. This is one of those breastfeeding myths. The nipples will toughen up as the baby nurses. Rolling or tugging at the nipple during pregnancy, or rubbing a rough towel on them was once thought to help, but now we know it doesn't really help. It might actually make them more tender. About the only thing you have to do is avoid using soap or alcohol on your nipples. Those products will wash away the nipples' natural oils. The key to preventing sore nipples is holding your baby in the correct position. If the baby is held correctly, latched on correctly, and sucking effectively, you shouldn't have a problem with sore nipples. Positioning is discussed in chapter 4.

To summarize, read all you can about breastfeeding, talk to women who have successfully breastfed, and maybe even take a breastfeeding class. Let your doctor (and also your baby's doctor) know you plan to breastfeed. The more you know before the baby arrives, the better prepared you will be.

Chapter Three

How the Breast Works

---

*It is hard to believe that my baby knows
exactly how much breast milk she needs. I just
feed her when she wants to nurse. I don't go
by the clock, but most days it is about every two
and a half hours. She is happy and I always seem
to have enough milk for her. I must be doing
something right. She is growing like a weed.*

Audra

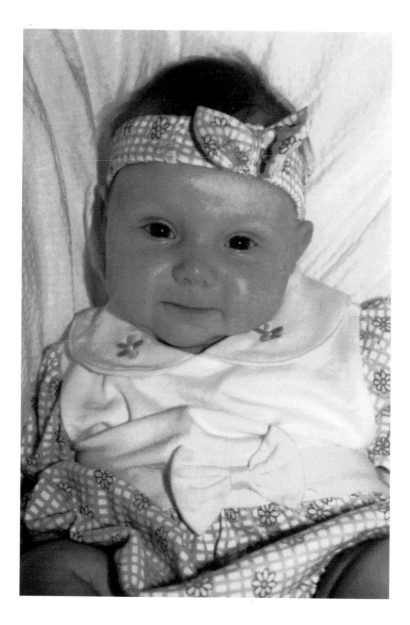

How The Breast Works

The lactating breast is remarkable, and will make all the milk a baby needs. Here's how:

When the baby sucks **correctly**, it causes the nerves, located underneath your **areola**, (the darker circle around the nipple) to tell the brain to release a hormone called **prolactin**. This hormone, in turn, signals the milk glands, located in the breast, to make milk. So, if a baby is sucking correctly and removing milk, *more milk will be produced*. When milk is *not* removed, milk production is decreased. That is why it is so important for the baby to suck effectively, and why it is important for the mother to nurse often during the first few weeks. It takes about six weeks for the milk supply to become well established.

The breast is made up of milk producing glands, ducts, and sinuses (reservoirs). The milk is made in the **milk glands** and then travels down the **duct** toward the nipple and is stored in the **sinus**. When the baby presses his jaw on the sinus, the milk comes out through the **nipple pores** into his mouth.

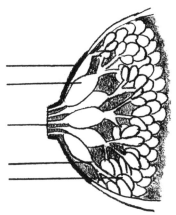

Areola
Milk sinus (reservoir)

Nipple pores

Milk duct
Milk producing gland

How the Baby Gets Milk

It takes a little effort for the baby to nurse. He must take the nipple far into the mouth, create a seal around the nipple and areola, compress the milk ducts with his jaws, move his tongue a certain way, and swallow.

You can see from the following diagram how the mother's nipple and breast tissue are formed into a "teat" and pulled far back into the mouth. The end of the nipple will touch the junction of the hard and soft palate, which will signal the baby to suckle. When the nipple is this far in, the jaws can compress (and "strip") the milk sinuses easily. The baby's tongue will be over the bottom gum (and any bottom teeth.) When the nipple is pulled into the baby's mouth correctly, and he suckles correctly, you will make plenty of milk and your nipples will not get sore.

Note: The extra effort involved in nursing will strengthen your baby's jaw and facial muscles, and may help prevent future speech and orthodontic problems.

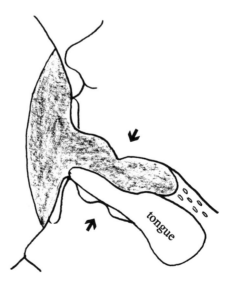

Correct latch-on. Notice how far the nipple goes into the mouth.

Another hormone, called **oxytocin**, causes the milk producing cells to release the milk into the ducts. When this happens, it is called the **let-down** or **milk ejection reflex.** Oxytocin is released when the baby suckles. It is also released at other times.

Sometimes you will have a let-down when you hear your baby cry, or if you're just thinking about him. Or you may have a let-down when you hear somebody else's baby cry! And sometimes let-downs even occur during sex. All these situations are normal and are usually temporary.

Oxytocin is a powerful hormone. It is the hormone that causes your uterus to contract, too. Sometimes mothers can feel these contractions (called after-pains) as the baby nurses. But these are temporary, also. You probably won't feel them after a few days.

For the first few weeks, while your breasts are adjusting, your breasts might feel "tingly" when your milk first lets down. Some mothers feel the sensation every time for the first few weeks, and others never feel it at all. Both situations are normal.

It sometimes takes a minute or so for the let-down to occur. When you notice your baby swallowing more often, or taking large gulps, you can be sure your milk has let down. Even though you may not feel each let-down happening, chances are you are having several at each feeding.

Over-active Letdowns

Some mothers have very forceful letdowns and the baby may choke and sputter. If this is a problem, take your baby off the breast for a moment and catch the milk in a towel (or a cup) before putting him back on. You might adjust him to a more upright posture, which may give him more control over the faster-flowing milk and thus reduce the choking. Or, you might try letting him nurse "upside down." Lie back in a recliner or bed and let the baby lie face down over your breast, as opposed to face-up under it. Just make sure he is latched on correctly.

Sometimes, if you have an over-abundance of milk, the let-downs can be forceful and the baby may choke or gag when he tries to nurse. Use the same measures as discussed above to control these letdowns. If forceful let-downs continue, and your baby fusses at the beginning of each feed, try nursing on only one side at each feeding. This helps to decrease the over-supply, and hopefully, the force of the let-down as well.

Foremilk and Hindmilk

Did you know there are two "kinds" of milk? Foremilk and hindmilk. *Foremilk* is the milk that has collected in the sinuses between feedings. It is thin and watery, and may even look a little blue. It is high in volume, but low in fat and calories.

As the baby nurses, the foremilk gradually is replaced by *hindmilk*. The amount of hindmilk is less than foremilk, but it is creamier and higher in fat and calories. Your baby needs hindmilk to gain weight sufficiently.

If your baby isn't gaining enough, he will need to nurse for longer lengths of time at each breast, so he will get plenty of the high-fat calories found in hindmilk.

Let the baby decide when he has had enough of the first breast. When he has had enough, he will come off the breast on his own. If he still appears hungry, then offer him the second breast. Let him nurse the second breast until he is thoroughly satisfied.

If you switch sides too soon, or too often, your baby

may get too much foremilk and not enough hindmilk. There must be a balance of the two types of milk. Your baby will know how much to take if you let him decide.

Sometimes, mothers have an overabundance of foremilk, and their babies get too much, causing an imbalance. These babies don't gain much weight and though they may be growing, they just never seem content. These babies want to nurse most of the time and cry a lot.

Greenish, frothy stools are another sign of foremilk/hindmilk imbalance. However, green stools do not always mean you have an imbalance problem. Sometimes the color just comes from what you have been eating. If your baby is content and gaining, green stools are not a problem.

Low Milk Supply

Occasionally a mom will have a low milk supply. She may think that everything is going right - she is nursing often, the baby is sucking correctly, but the baby is not gaining or may be crying a lot. If you want to increase your milk supply, there are several things you can do.

- Get plenty of rest. Plan to take a couple of days off and concentrate on your milk supply. Take your baby to bed with you, get lots of skin-to-skin contact and nurse, nurse, nurse!

- Nurse often, for at least 20 minutes at each feeding. Nurse from both breasts so they will both get stimulation.

- If you are using formula, cut back gradually. Don't use any pacifiers or nipple shields.

- There are some medications that are prescribed to increase milk supply. Discuss this with your doctor or lactation consultant.

- Some women also find it helps to take herbs and herb teas to increase milk supply. A good lactation consultant may be able to recommend which ones to use or seek help from a knowledgeable health food store employee. Some grocery stores carry "Mother's Milk Tea" which helps some mothers.

There are some women who just don't make enough milk to completely sustain their babies, but it is very rare (probably less than 5% of all women). These women may not have had noticeable breast changes during pregnancy and they may not have breast changes after the baby's birth. This could be genetic; it could come from surgeries, or it could come from other traumas to the breasts which might be interfering with milk production; or they might have hormonal imbalances interfering with either milk production or let-down. Mothers who truly have insufficient milk will have to supplement with donor human milk or formula.

Chapter Four

In the Hospital

I got to nurse my baby right after he was born. The nurse laid him on my chest and after squirming around a little bit, he found my nipple and latched right on! It was great. Even the doctor was amazed at how quickly he caught on. He nursed from then on whenever he needed to, and I didn't have any problems.

Jennifer

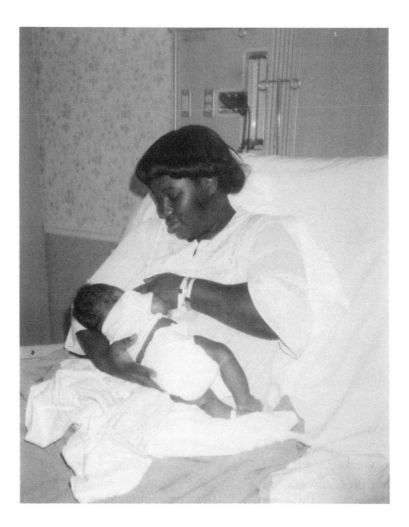

In The Hospital

The first few feedings are very important. The sooner you nurse, the better for you and the baby. Newborns are very alert and calm for the first couple of hours after birth, and if your baby is like most, he won't have any trouble latching on immediately after birth. However, there are newborns who are not interested in nursing at first. Some are too medicated from the mother's labor medications and may only nuzzle, or lick the breast or just want to sleep. Whether your baby actually nurses or not the first time, it will still be a very special time for you and your baby. It is the beginning of bonding.

But bonding is not the only benefit to nursing immediately after birth. The sooner you put the baby to breast, and the more often you nurse, thereafter, the more milk-making cells will be developed. The sucking will also stimulate the uterus to contract and help control any bleeding.

Be sure and tell your doctor or midwife ahead of time that you want to nurse as soon as possible after birth, preferably immediately after birth, but definitely within the first hour. Your baby's first bath can wait!

Colostrum

Colostrum is the first milk an infant receives from the breast. It is thick and yellow, and is loaded with proteins and antibodies that are essential to your baby's health. Your body knows exactly what your baby needs. For instance, if he is born early, the colostrum will have factors which are more suitable for a preterm baby. Or if he is born into an environment where there are certain illnesses present, colostrum will have antibodies in it to counter those illnesses. It is truly a "wonder" food. Lucky is the child who receives his own mother's colostrum.

Colostrum has a laxative effect, and helps rid the baby's body of meconium, the waste product produced in the womb. The quick elimination of meconium will help prevent him from becoming jaundiced.

In some cultures, it is believed that colostrum is "bad" and mothers are told to wait a few days before nursing. This belief is simply *not true*. It is very important that your baby gets your colostrum. (To give you an example of how important colostrum is in another mammal: Most calves *die* when deprived of their mother's colostrum, and farmers do all they can to make sure calves get it.)

When the Milk "Comes In"

The more you nurse, the quicker your milk will change from colostrum to mature milk. It usually takes about 2 or 3 days for your milk to "come in." If you have had a Cesarean section, or a large blood loss, it might take a few days longer. Most new mothers worry about their milk coming in. They may have heard that their breasts will be engorged, and that they will be very uncomfortable, and some even worry that their milk won't come in at all.

If your baby has nursed often since his birth, (at least every 2-3 hours) your milk *will* come in, and you probably won't have a problem with undue engorgement (swelling). Severe engorgement can occur when the baby isn't nursing often enough, or if the breasts are not being emptied.

If for some reason, your breasts do get swollen and tender, it is best to nurse often, and use a breast pump, or hand express before feedings to make latch-on easier, or after feedings to make sure the breasts are emptied. Before a feeding, massaging the breasts with warm, wet cloths, or massaging while standing in a warm shower will help the milk flow. Or if a mother is abundantly endowed, she might lean over a basin of warm water, letting her breasts float in the warm water.

Motrin or Tylenol might help with the discomfort while waiting for the other remedies to relieve the engorgement itself.

Engorgement and Cabbage Leaves???

If you are really engorged and uncomfortable, and warm showers and Motrin haven't helped, try the CABBAGE LEAF treatment.

Although it might sound bizarre, it is a remedy that often works. No one really knows why, but it is thought that there are substances in cabbage leaves (absorbed through the skin) that help reduce swelling. Many hospital maternity units now keep cabbage leaves on hand for engorgement.

Here's how:

- Place CLEAN, refrigerated, outer CABBAGE LEAVES on your breasts (cover completely, down to the armpits). Some lactation consultants recommend rolling the leaves with a rolling pin to break the veins in the leaves.

- Cover the cabbage leaves with cool, wet cloths and leave on for about 15 minutes. Lying down makes it easier.

- After removing the leaves, massage the breasts and put warm, wet cloths on them.

- Nurse or pump after treatment.

- Repeat several times a day, but don't over-do it, because constant application of cabbage leaves may reduce milk production.

Cabbage leaves may also be used to relieve isolated packed or tender engorged areas of the breast or underarms. Place cold leaves against just the affected area, and watch the swelling disappear!

Sometimes a breast is so swollen that the nipple "flattens out" and the baby can't latch on correctly. If this happens, massage, then express or pump out a little milk before you try to nurse the baby. Since sore nipples can be caused by incorrect latching, it is important to soften the nipple area before you try latching.

Remember, nursing often from birth should prevent severe engorgement. But if it happens, don't give up on nursing. It WILL get better. Engorgement is very temporary. It probably won't last more than a day or so.

Positioning your Baby

How you hold your baby is very important. If he is not positioned just right, your nipples can get sore. Because the nerves (located under the areola area) in the nipple might not get enough stimulation, and the milk sinuses are not adequately compressed, you might not produce enough milk. To make any position work best, bring baby's head and mouth to the nipple (as opposed to moving breast and nipple to the baby). Baby's body should be facing mom's and as much as possible, baby's arms should be around mom's breast, not between baby and breast.

There are several ways to position your baby. The most common way is called the **cradle or Madonna hold.**

• First, make yourself comfortable. Sit in a comfortable chair (use a footstool if you are short) or prop yourself in bed with several pillows.

• Rest the baby's head on your forearm, directly facing your breast. His body should be facing you. (Never have the baby's head turned and his body facing upward. This makes it hard for him to swallow.) His back should be supported by your arm and his bottom held up with your hand. Hold the baby **level** with your breast and don't lean forward. Move your baby, not your breast, to get a good alignment. You might have to use a pillow on your lap to help support him.

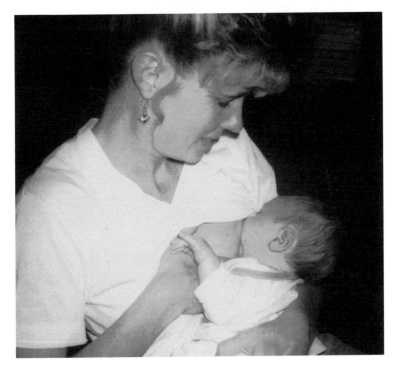

Cradle Hold

- Tickle his lip with your nipple, and wait for him to open his mouth **wide**. (Hint: If you open *your* mouth wide, he may mimic you and open his.)

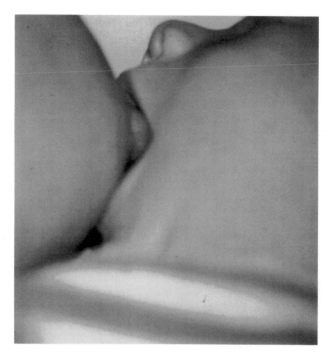

Wait until baby opens wide.

- When his mouth is wide open, quickly pull him to your breast so that the chin touches the breast first. He should now "latch on" to the breast just right. The lower lip should be as far from the base of the nipple as possible and you should be able to see some of the areola above the top lip. If he is not positioned just right, take him off and start over.

If you have a Cesarean section, you can still nurse in the

cradle hold position. Have the nurse help you prop up in bed and use lots of pillows. To protect your incision, use a pillow in your lap for the baby to lie on.

Lying Down to Nurse

Many mothers who have had Cesareans are often more comfortable, or find it easier, using a **side-lying** position. Have the nurse help you turn over on your side and lay the baby facing your breast. Follow the same steps as outlined for the cradle hold, but place him on his side and facing you. You might put a pillow behind him to help keep him in place. And putting pillows behind *your* back to support your weight will make you more comfortable. The baby's head may either be on your arm or on the bed, whichever is more comfortable.

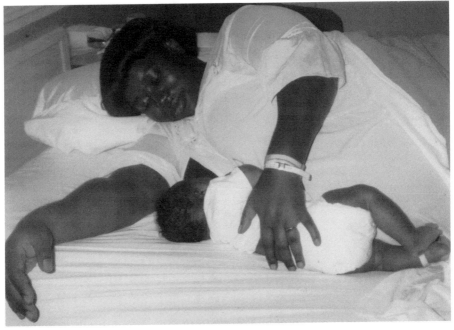

Lying down to nurse

Clutch Hold (Football)

Other mothers who have had Cesareans prefer the **clutch (football) hold.** This is also a good position for dealing with over-active let-downs, to help sleepy babies become more alert, or to encourage babies to open jaws wider. This is also a good way to nurse twins simultaneously.

• Hold the baby on your arm with his feet toward your back. His head should be supported by your hand.

• Tickle his lips and as soon as he opens wide, pull him to the breast, making sure the chin touches the breast first.

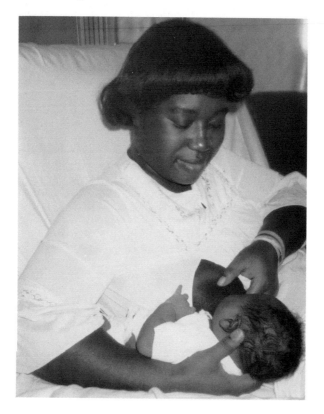

Football hold

Across-the-lap Hold

There is one other position, called the **across-the-lap hold**. In this position the baby is held across the lap, like the cradle hold, but in the opposite arm to the breast being used. Baby's body lies along your forearm, still turned towards you, but his head is now supported by your hand rather than the bend in your elbow. The other hand either supports the breast or his head. Some moms may find it a little harder to keep the baby close enough to the breast in this position.

Across-the-lap hold

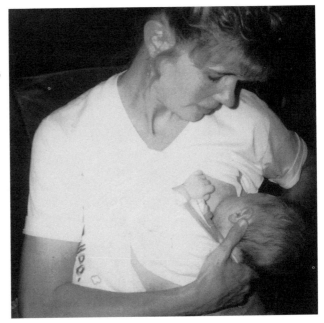

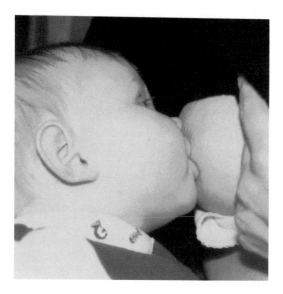

Notice how both lips are flanged out.

Again, understand, no matter what position you use, a baby must be latched on correctly. The chin must be tucked in close, and some of the areola must be showing above the top lip. **The top and bottom lips should both be flanged out.** His tongue should be well over his bottom gum.

Sucking Problems

If your baby's cheeks seem to be sunk in (instead of rounded), or if he keeps coming off the breast, or if you hear "clicking" or slurping sounds while he eats, your baby may have a sucking problem.

Occasionally babies just can't quite suck correctly. Sucking problems may be a result of medicines mom received prior to or during labor and delivery. They may be due to birth trauma, or may even be a result of sucking habits already developed in utero.

A baby may suck his tongue, or use his tongue incorrectly. If he was sucking against his fist in utero, he may not want the nipple and areola adequately in his mouth, or if he sucked his finger in utero, he may not want to open his mouth wide enough. Or he may be quite happy to suck on his own tongue or upper lip, and this makes it hard for him to nurse correctly.

Sucking problems usually mean the baby is not stimulating the nipple area enough to establish a good milk supply, and he is probably not getting enough milk. Sucking problems can be serious, but it does not mean you have to put your baby on a bottle.

Almost all sucking problems are transitory and will improve with time, patience, practice, and the help of trained personnel. A good lactation consultant will be able to identify the problem and help you teach your baby to latch on and nurse correctly.

How To Get the Baby Off the Breast

It is always better to let the baby decide when he is finished. You will know, because he will either fall asleep, or be so satisfied that he comes off the breast by himself. However, if for some reason you want to end the nursing session, or want to switch sides, just stick a clean finger in the corner of his mouth, between the gums, to break the suction. Pulling the baby off without breaking the suction first can damage your nipple.

After-pains

For the first few days after childbirth, you might notice more bleeding (lochia) as you nurse. This is normal. As the uterus contracts and curls up, it presses out blood that has collected in the uterus. You might feel your uterus contracting (cramping) while the baby nurses. Some mothers feel the "after-pains," others don't. Usually with the first pregnancy, moms don't feel these cramps, or feel them only mildly or briefly. With subsequent babies, the uterus must work harder to close down, as it is more stretched out, and moms might feel the cramping more severely. If the cramps really hurt, ask for a painkiller about a half hour before nursing. Both the cramping and the increased bleeding with nursing are normal. They mean that your body and uterus are doing their proper job, and the total childbirth process is being completed.

Rooming In

You and your baby will get off to a better start if you choose "rooming-in." This means the baby is allowed to stay in your room instead of the nursery. Most hospitals have that option now. It allows you to care for your baby, and nurse whenever he needs to, day or night. It is a wonderful way to get breastfeeding off to a good start. Hospitals that are "baby friendly" allow rooming-in, and encourage you to nurse on demand. There are often lactation consultants in these hospitals who will help you to breastfeed successfully.

Rooming-in also helps the new family to bond. Many of the hospitals that have rooming-in now also allow the father and siblings unlimited visits.

Chapter Five

The First Few Weeks

Coming home with my new baby was the happiest day of my life. My mother came and stayed the first few days which helped a lot. She did the cooking and cleaning and let me tend to my daughter. Nursing was a little hard the first few weeks, but it got much easier as time went by. I wouldn't want to feed my child any other way!

Pattie

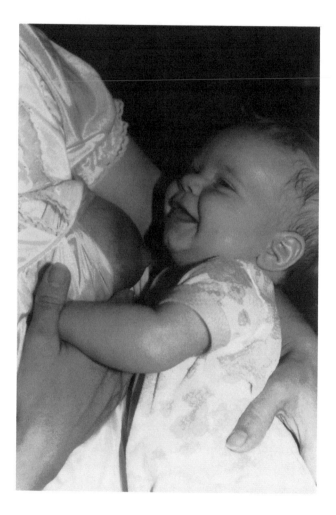

Unless there are complications, you won't be in the hospital very long. Today, many hospitals are sending mothers and babies home in 24 hours (some even less) and that doesn't give you much time to adjust to breastfeeding. That is why it is so important you have a supportive husband, friend, or relative around to help. And having the phone number of a La Leche League Leader or lactation consultant might really come in handy.

The following paragraphs will tell you how and when to nurse your baby:

The First Few Days

Mothers who are breastfeeding are now being encouraged and taught to feed their breastfed infants on "demand," which means you feed the baby whenever he wants to nurse. However, this *does not* apply to the first 2 or 3 days of a baby's life, because some babies just don't "demand" to be fed often enough. Many are too sleepy and uninterested. (Note: Some childbirth medications cause babies to sleep too long or to have difficulty nursing effectively.)

Because your baby may be too sleepy and uninterested those first couple of days, you may have to waken him to nurse. He MUST nurse at least every 2-3 hours those first few days. One 4-6 hour stretch is acceptable in a 24 hour time-period, but ONLY IF baby has been eating at least every two hours, correctly and effectively the rest of the time. Doing this will ensure that your baby gets your valuable colostrum and will promote milk production. By all means, wake your baby up if he sleeps as long as three hours. And try to keep him awake at the breast. Loosening or removing his clothing, burping, or massaging him will help. Be gentle but insistent. He MUST nurse at least every 2-3 hours those first few days. It doesn't happen often, but some babies become dehydrated if they are not nursed often and long enough those first few days. Signs of dehydration are discussed in the next chapter.

Nursing On Demand

After the first few days you should nurse your baby "on demand" or "on cue." That means you feed him when he gives you signals that he NEEDS to nurse. It will probably be very sporadic for a while, and you may feel like you are nursing all the time. This is normal.

Babies, first of all, have very small tummies. Secondly, breastmilk is digested much more easily, more completely, and much faster than formula, so your baby won't go nearly as long between feedings as a bottle baby. Even when babies eat every 2-3 hours, babies will need, take, and be satisfied with, far less volume of breastmilk than they would of formula. This is due both to the composition of breastmilk, and to the way it "lets down."

Relax and don't look at the clock. If he nurses for 20 minutes, falls asleep and then wakes up again 30 minutes later, wanting to nurse, then go ahead and nurse him again. This is entirely normal for the adjustment period. In a few weeks, as your milk supply builds up, and he learns to nurse more efficiently, your baby will go much longer between feedings, and might even get into a regular routine of eating every two to three hours. He might even sleep an occasional stretch of five to six hours. If you're really lucky, this sleep stretch will happen at night.

You will soon learn to recognize your baby's hunger signals. He will start to fuss, squirm, chew his fists or "root" (looking for the breast). Don't wait until he starts to scream. By that time, he will be so upset and hungry that he won't be able to settle down and nurse calmly. Or he may nurse so vigorously that he hurts your nipples.

When a baby cries, he has a need. It may be that he is hot, cold, wet, hungry or just lonesome. If he can't be comforted any other way than nursing, then he **needs** to nurse. You can't over-feed a breastfed baby. He will stop when he has enough.

Burping Your Baby

Breastfed babies don't swallow as much air as bottle-fed babies. However, you might try to burp him after he comes off the first breast. If he hasn't burped in a minute or two, he probably doesn't need to.

Some babies who are not burped during feedings, "feel" full, and fall asleep at the breast before getting enough. This could affect the milk supply and the baby's weight. Burping usually makes babies want to nurse a while longer.

How Long to Feed

Do you time the feedings, or do you let the baby decide? Correct answer: Let the baby decide.

Don't watch the clock. Watch your baby. Let him nurse the first breast until he stops sucking. If your breast is soft and he falls asleep or seems content, he is probably satisfied. But if he doesn't seem entirely satisfied, try switching to the other side. He should then nurse the second breast until he is fully content. At the next feeding, start with the side you stopped on. It will probably feel heavier.

Some women prefer to nurse on only one breast at each feeding. This can work, also. It will take about thirty minutes. Babies usually get more of the high-fat creamy milk when they nurse one breast at a feeding, and often gain more weight.

Your baby is smart. He knows exactly how much milk he *needs*, and which kind (foremilk or hindmilk.) If he *needs* the high calorie hindmilk, he will want to nurse a long time at each breast. If he just *needs* to quench his thirst (maybe on a hot day), he may nurse frequently but for shorter periods, getting the more plentiful and watery, low fat milk. Let your baby be the boss, and he will get exactly what he needs from each breast.

Baby's Bowel Movements

The first few bowel movements of a breastfed baby will be black, tarry-looking and sticky. This is meconium. It is made of hair, skin cells, and vernix (the white coating babies are born with) that baby has shed during the pregnancy, and which has been filtered out of the amniotic fluid (bag of waters) into the baby's gut. It also contains bilirubin, which is excreted into the baby's bowel from his kidney.

If a baby doesn't have a lot of bowel movements in the first few days, this bilirubin will be reabsorbed into the baby's blood stream, and may cause him to become jaundiced. Since colostrum has a slightly laxative effect we encourage moms to breastfeed often to keep the meconium moving. This will help to minimize or decrease the jaundice that might develop from having too few bowel movements.

The next bowel movements are called transitional stool. This may be greenish and watery-looking, with what looks like seeds or curds lying in it. Sometimes parents think the baby is having diarrhea, but it isn't. Diarrhea smells bad, or foul while the transitional stools continue to have the same "sweetish" smell that the meconium had.

As your milk comes in, those seedy stools will turn more yellow or tan. They are usually soft and semi-formed (about the consistency of yogurt or cottage cheese), and they continue to have a slightly sweet smell. Sometimes, because they are so soft, moms again think the baby has diarrhea. But he probably doesn't. Again, diarrhea usually has a very bad smell, one that is quite different than the odor of a formula fed or partially formula fed baby.

While some babies have a little bowel movement after every feeding, after three or four days, most babies have at least 2 "substantial" bowel movements a day. Whether it's a lot of little bowel movements or 2 or 3 big ones a day, it is normal for a breastfed baby. Because breastmilk is so well digested, a completely breastfed baby probably will not get constipated.

Note: After the first six weeks or so, your baby may go several days without a bowel movement. Don't be concerned, he is probably not constipated. In fact, your older baby may go as long as 5-7 days without a bowel movement and show no signs of being uncomfortable. (Warning: When he does decide to go, watch out! It will be a big, messy one.)

One more thing. It is normal for some breastfed babies to grunt and strain or cry during bowel movements, but as long as they are on breastmilk only, they are not constipated.

Mother's Biggest Worry

Many mothers worry that their baby is not getting enough milk. And it can be especially worrisome if your friends and relatives (and even your spouse) are making comments like, "Are you SURE he is getting enough breast milk?" or "He just fed 2 hours ago. You must not have enough milk!" People who say things like this have probably never nursed a baby, and probably know very little about it. Ignore them. Try to educate them and follow these guidelines:

How to tell if your baby is getting enough:

- Your baby is breastfeeding effectively at least 10-12 times in 24 hours.

- He is content, alert, and gaining at a *steady* pace. Note: It is normal for babies to lose a few ounces the first few days but they should regain the lost ounces by 2 weeks.

- When he sucks, you see his jaws moving in a steady rhythm, and after every 2-3 sucks, you see him pause as he swallows a mouthful of milk. You may hear him swallow.

- You see milk pooling in your baby's mouth when he comes off the breast.

- Your breasts feel softer and lighter at the end of each feeding.

- Beginning the third or fourth day, he is having at least 6-8 soaking wet diapers in a 24 hour period. (It's normal if your baby has only 1-2 wet diapers the first day or two.) The color of the urine should be pale. If you use disposable diapers, it may be hard to tell when they are wet. Putting a strip of tissue in the diaper will help you tell.

- Your baby is having a little bowel movement after the end of every feeding or at least 2 very large bowel movements in each 24 hour period.

Sometimes, (but rarely) a mother just doesn't make enough milk for her baby. A poor milk supply is usually caused by not nursing often enough, or by nursing incorrectly. Nursing more often, especially during the night, and making sure that the baby is latched on and sucking effectively will often solve the problem.

Even more rare (thought to be less than 5 percent of women) is the woman who has insufficient glandular tissue in the breast. This may be suspected when the breasts have not grown larger during pregnancy or if the milk didn't appear to "come in" the first week. If you are really worried that your baby is not getting enough breastmilk, then you must watch him carefully for signs of dehydration.

Your baby may be dehydrated if:

- he acts listless and sick
- his urine is a dark yellow color
- his mouth and lips are dry
- the soft spot (fontanel) on the top of his head sinks in.

All of these symptoms are serious. Take your baby to a doctor *immediately* if he has any of them.

Breast Compression

During the first few weeks, babies often fall asleep at the breast when the flow of milk is slow, and they may not be getting enough. Breast compression is one way of making sure your baby gets what he needs. It simulates a let-down and sometimes even stimulates an actual let-down. Breast compression may be done when the baby isn't gaining adequately, or if he seems to want to nurse "all the time," or is colicky. It is also useful if a mother has recurrent blocked ducts and mastitis.

Breast compression continues the flow of milk when the baby starts to fall asleep and results in the baby getting more milk, especially the hindmilk.

Here is how to do breast compression:

- Hold the baby in one arm. Hold the breast with the other hand, with the thumb on one side and your fingers on the other side, fairly far away from the nipple.

- Watch your baby. When he stops drinking and is just "nibbling," compress your breast. Do not press hard enough to hurt yourself.

- Keep the pressure up until the baby is no longer drinking and then release the pressure. The baby will start sucking when the milk starts to flow again.

- Continue on the first side until the baby does not drink even with the compression. If he wants more, repeat with the second side.

- Remember, do not compress hard enough to hurt. As the baby gets more efficient at nursing and/or latch-on improves, you will not have to continue breast compression.

(Breast Compression instructions adapted from handout by Jack Newman, MD, FRCPC)

Supplementing With Formula and Giving Water

Breastmilk has all the nutrients your breastfed baby needs and supplementing with formula is sometimes risky. If your baby isn't gaining, you may need a lactation consultant to do a suck evaluation. Or you may just need to nurse more often, or start nursing on only one side at each feeding so that the baby gets more of the rich hindmilk.

At the first checkup, your baby will be weighed. And if the doctor thinks the baby isn't gaining adequately, he may prescribe formula. You have the right to question the doctor about this, and to explore other options. **Even one bottle of** formula a day can be detrimental to your baby's health and your milk supply. Here's why:

- You think your baby needs more milk, so you give him a bottle of formula.

- Your baby gets thoroughly satiated and sleeps 3-4 hours, missing a breastfeeding session.

- Your breasts begin to make less milk because they did not receive the signal to make more milk.

- When you nurse the next time, your baby gets fussy because there isn't as much milk.

- You feed him a little more formula. Your breasts make even less milk.

- Now your baby isn't nursing nearly as often, and you are making less milk. You *have* to feed him formula.

- Soon your baby will be completely off the breast and drinking formula, which is **INFERIOR** in every way!

Remember, the more milk that is removed, the more milk you will make. And if you fill the baby up with formula, he will nurse less, and you won't make as much milk. There is nothing better for your baby than breastmilk.

Water is *not* necessary for a completely breastfed baby, even in hot climates. Giving babies water to hold them to the next feeding has the effect of diluting the food they are getting, be it breastmilk or formula. Further, it can cause problems with the baby's electrolyte balance, which is the balance of many of the body's chemical elements. And finally, it can cause problems, especially in the early weeks, with proper closure of the linings of the infant's intestines. The recent American Academy of Pediatrics Breastfeeding Policy Statement states "no supplements (water, glucose water, formula, and so forth) should be given to breastfeeding newborns unless a medical indication exists." *(Pediatrics, December,1997)*

Giving bottles of anything, water, formula, or even breastmilk, in the first few weeks of life, may lead to another problem - nipple confusion or preference.

Nipple Confusion/Preference

Sucking on a synthetic nipple is very different than sucking at the mother's breast. There is a different taste and texture. A baby must work his tongue and jaws much differently to bottle-feed than to breastfeed. He must learn to coordinate breathing and swallowing differently in the two different types of eating. And finally, the availability of milk, and the flow-rate differ from bottle to breast.

Some babies very quickly develop a preference for the bottle - the milk comes instantly, and it is much easier for him. In bottlefeeding, the baby has to do very little except react to the flow of milk. After a few bottles, they may seem to "forget" how to nurse. And some babies, especially if they still aren't sucking effectively, may get confused about "how to eat," because "how to eat" keeps changing from one meal to the next.

If your baby is actually nipple confused, he CAN still learn to breastfeed. If he has developed a preference, and is refusing the breast, he CAN be re-taught. Keep "working" at breastfeeding, and take away all bottles and pacifiers. If he won't nurse at all, pump your breasts and feed him breastmilk with an eyedropper, spoon, cup or nursing supplementer. Most of the time, after a couple of days of effort, he will get back on the breast. But if he doesn't, don't give up. Ask for help from your lactation consultant or LLL Leader. They will soon have your baby nursing again.

Pacifiers

Pacifiers are another cause of developing nipple preference or confusion. While there may be rare times when you have to use one, you shouldn't rely on one very often. If your baby is given a pacifier every time he fusses, he may not nurse enough to keep up your milk supply, and he may not gain enough weight. Your milk supply *may be affected*. And pacifiers can also affect the way teeth grow in.

If you have extremely sore nipples, or if you are somewhere where you just *can't* nurse, you may have to use a pacifier temporarily. Holding the baby when he is using a pacifier is better than putting him down with it.

Some babies will refuse to take a pacifier. They don't want "second best" and just won't take one. Do you blame them? And some babies will take one kind and not another. You might have to experiment with several different types before you find one your baby will take.

Remember, a pacifier can be useful at certain times, but it may affect your milk supply in the early weeks. It can cause nipple confusion and it is very habit-forming. Babies hooked on pacifiers will not give them up easily. It is best not to use pacifiers at all.

Note: Recent research (*Lancet*, April 1996) shows that pacifier use may be linked to lower IQ, and may, in fact, account for some of the IQ deficits noted in bottle-fed infants.

Sleeping Through the Night

Motherhood is not easy. Babies have to be fed, changed, rocked, and they generally require almost constant attention. Even at night. And many mothers wonder when (or if) their babies will *ever* sleep through the night.

All babies are different, and so are their sleeping habits. Some sleep through the night at 2 weeks, and others don't until they are 2 or 3 years old. Most bottle-fed babies don't sleep all night either for a while. But most babies will sleep for longer periods of time as time goes on.

For the first few weeks, your breastfed baby will need to nurse during the night. It will be better for him and for you. Breastmilk is digested very quickly, and he will probably get hungry several times during the night. This is normal. Breastfeeding during the night also helps keep up your milk supply, and keeps you from becoming engorged.

Although sleeping through the night is seen as an "accomplishment," a goal to be achieved as early as possible, it really shouldn't be seen that way. It is normal for children to wake at night for the first several years. If you realize this and know that sleeping deeply for long stretches of time can be dangerous for infants (because of the risk of SIDS) your baby's night waking will not seem to be such an inconvenience. Your own sleep patterns will change and you will get used to it. If you have your baby in bed with you, neither of you has to fully wake up to nurse. Soon you won't even be disturbed by the baby waking up and eating. You might even half-sleep right through it.

Some babies sleep through the night for a while, and then when they start teething, they start waking up again. When they are in pain, they can't sleep, and nursing will help them get back to sleep.

Other people might suggest to you to feed cereal or

formula to your baby at bedtime to sleep through. This is not really a good idea. Your baby's digestive system may not be able to handle it yet, or he may actually be allergic to the proteins in formula and cereal. There are studies that have shown that feeding cereal at bedtime doesn't really work, anyway, to make babies sleep longer.

Don't worry if your baby is not sleeping through the night yet. He WILL eventually sleep all night.

Growth Spurts

Most babies go through periods of sudden growth during the early months, and they will want to nurse more often during these times. Some days it may seem like he wants to nurse every hour. You are not losing your milk. He is just going through a growth spurt.

Growth spurts only last a day or two, just long enough for the baby to build up your milk supply enough to meet his growing needs. Just knowing about growth spurts will help you when the time comes.

The first growth spurt will come around the 10th to 14th day. This is also about the time you notice that your breasts aren't as full as they once were. This is normal. You still have your milk, only the swelling has gone down. The more frequent nursings will help you make even more milk.

The second growth spurt comes around 4 to 6 weeks. By this time, your baby is growing at a very fast rate. After a day or two of nursing marathons, he will be feeding normally.

"Spoiling" the Baby

Crying is the newborn's way of communicating. When he cries, he has a need. He may be hungry, wet, too hot, too cold, scared, bored, need burping, or just need to be held.

Whatever the reason, it is a *need*.

Your baby wants and needs to feel you close by, and if he stops crying when you pick him up and cuddle him, then that is what he needs. The sound of your heartbeat, the warmth of your arms, your voice, your smell, and the rhythm of your breathing are all comforting to your baby.

There are some babies who seem to need to be held most of the time. They are sometimes referred to as "high-need" babies and life can get pretty difficult if you have one. It gets especially hard if you have other children in the family. Some mothers use a carrier or sling that allows them to "wear" their babies while they do other things, and these devices seem to help a great deal. The baby stays close to the mother, and feels very secure. He cries much less.

You can't "spoil" a newborn baby. Babies are meant to be held and loved. And who can resist picking up a newborn, when he so desperately wants to be picked up? If you don't meet your child's needs while he is a baby, he may have more serious emotional problems later.

All babies cry, but it is not a good idea to let him cry long and hard. Studies have shown that hard crying in the early days of a newborn's life can lead to problems with the baby's heart or bleeding in the brain.

A baby who is cared for and loved will learn to love and trust his parents and will grow up to love and trust others. He will feel secure, and be able to adjust to life's problems.

Don't worry about spoiling your baby. Enjoy him while you can, and *listen to your heart*. Breastfeeding is the natural way to provide both the nutritional and emotional needs of your baby.

Nursing Away From Home

Babies don't always want to nurse at convenient times and places. You might find yourself having to nurse away from home at times, and you may feel shy or embarrassed about it. You may get over those feelings as time goes by. But, in the meantime, learning to nurse *discreetly* will help you to nurse more comfortably in less private surroundings.

Over the shoulder slings allow moms to nurse easily and comfortably and still see their babies as they nurse, without "baring all." Or, moms may find if sufficient to drape a shawl or blanket around their shoulders and their baby, letting the baby nurse without being exposed to the public eye. This can sometimes be arranged in such a way to still allow eye-contact between mom and baby.

What you wear makes a big difference. Most mothers find that overblouses and sweaters work best. Just lift up your blouse from the bottom, and tuck the baby in. You can also cover yourself with blankets and shawls. If you wear a button-up blouse, be sure to unbutton from the bottom instead of the top, so your breasts will be covered. And wearing a two-piece dress with a half slip is great for dress-up occasions. When you wear a three piece outfit (skirt or pants, blouse & jacket) no one will ever guess when you are nursing.

Dresses can be modified for nursing by sewing in zippers or velcro under tucks or darts, and there are patterns designed just for nursing mothers. There are several companies that specialize in fashions for the nursing mom. They sell clothes that are stylish and made so that no one knows about the "secret" openings. Refer to the appendix of this book for a list of these catalog companies.

It takes a little practice to learn to nurse discreetly, but you can do it. Nurse in front of a mirror before your first trip out and try on several outfits until you find one that allows you to nurse discreetly.

You will no doubt want to take your baby with you on outings, so here are some suggestions that will help:

- In restaurants, ask for a booth near the back of the room, or sit facing away from other people.

- In shopping malls or stores, ask to use a dressing room. Or if necessary, go sit in your car a few minutes. Please don't use public rest rooms, unless they are clean and spacious, or at least have an area to sit down that is not a toilet stall. Would you want to eat *your* lunch in a bathroom?

- If you are in someone else's home, and you feel uncomfortable breastfeeding in front of your hosts, their families or other guests, ask where you might have some privacy. If you sense that breastfeeding openly might make *them* uncomfortable, you might ask the same thing.

Don't fret about being harassed about breastfeeding in public. In many states you are actually protected by laws that prevent harassment. People *need* to see more mothers breastfeeding. It needs to be just as acceptable to breastfeed in public as to bottle-feed. And the more women who do it, the more acceptable it will be in time.

Other mothers who are nursing, or mothers who have nursed previously are always thrilled to see another mother who is unafraid to meet her child's need. These women are likely to give you a smile or a thumbs-up signal when they see you nursing in a public place!

Relax, enjoy your baby, and nurse him whenever he needs to nurse. With practice, you will soon be nursing comfortably, discreetly or openly, anytime and anywhere.

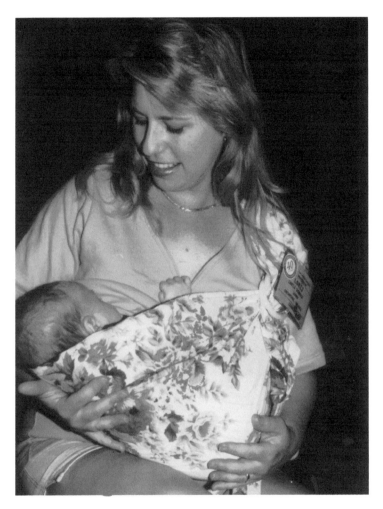

Nursing Discreetly

Chapter Six

Breastfeeding Gadgets

---

*I received all sorts of breastfeeding equipment
at my baby shower. I used breast pads for a few days
and I used a breast pump a few times when I knew
I was going out. But I really didn't need many
"things" to help me breastfeed. Nursing is
supposed to be natural, and thankfully, it was
for me.*

Maureen

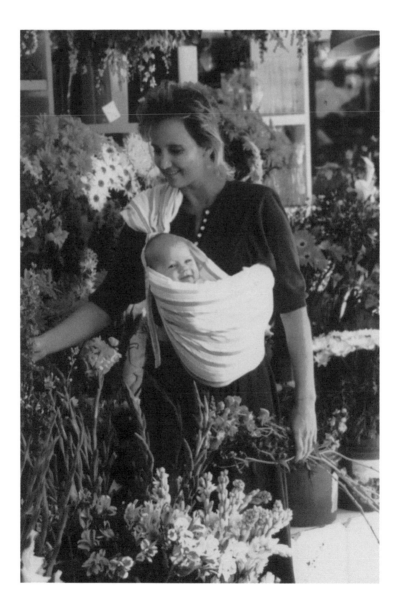

Breastfeeding Gadgets

There are all sorts of breastfeeding "gadgets" on the market these days. Everything from breast pumps to special bras are sold as "necessities" for breastfeeding mothers.

While some of these items are useful at times, most are not necessary for breastfeeding. Remember, mothers have been nursing their babies successfully since the beginning of time without ANY breastfeeding aids. Here are some of the items marketed to breastfeeding mothers.

BREAST PUMPS

Breast pumps are nice to have on hand, but unless you are going to be separated from your child for long lengths of time, they are not necessary. If you only need to express your milk occasionally, learning to hand-express may be best for you. Hand expression is discussed in chapter twelve.

Breast pumps are used by mothers who, for one reason or another, must be separated from the baby, but who still want the baby to receive breastmilk. Sometimes the mother or the baby may be hospitalized, or sometimes the mother may simply want to leave the baby for a few hours. And many times pumps are used by working mothers who want to leave breastmilk while they are at work.

Hand Pumps

There are many different hand pumps on the market today. The most common hand pump is probably the **cylinder** type. It looks like two tubes (usually made of clear plastic), one of which fits inside the other. It creates a vacuum (suction) when the inner tube is pulled in and out. The milk goes directly into the outer tube or into a standard bottle. It is easy to use and is convenient to carry with you. It is also easy to clean. There are several brands on the market and most work about the same. The White River brand features a flexible shield which some mothers say helps stimulate milk production.

Ameda Egnell makes a pump that can be operated with one hand. The design of this pump allows the mother to pump while nursing.

White River's Cylinder Pump →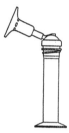

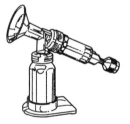 ← *Medela's Manual Pump*

Ameda-Egnell's One-Hand Pump →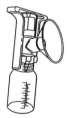

Small Battery Operated/Electric Pumps

Another type of pump is the small battery operated pump. They are small and can be used with one hand. Medela's Mini-Electric has automatic rhythmic suction, but most do not. The biggest complaint about battery operated pumps is the short life span of the batteries. However, most can be converted to electricity with the use of an adapter. They are much more efficient when used with an adapter. Small battery/electric pumps are only recommended for short term, occasional use. If you have a preemie who must remain in the hospital a long time or if you plan to pump at work, you will need a more substantial pump. But if you only need a pump occasionally these pumps will do just fine.

Medela's Mini-Electric →

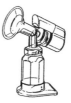

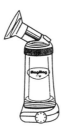

← *Omron's Mag-Mag pump*

Gerber pump →

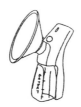

Medium-Sized Electric Pumps

If you are going back to work, there are several **medium-size electric breast pumps** available for that purpose. Two breast pump manufacturers, (Bailey, Medela) now have affordably priced electric pumps that are portable and lightweight. Some working mothers prefer to purchase a good pump instead of renting one. All these pumps have double kits included that allow you to pump both breasts at once. They all come in carrying cases and are convenient to take to work.

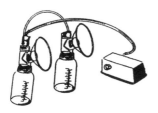

← *Bailey's Nurture III*

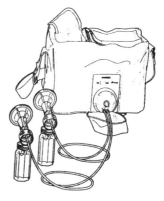

Medela's Pump-in-Style →

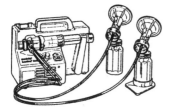

← *Medela's Lactina can be purchased or rented.*

Hospital-Grade Electric Pumps

For long-term pumping, you will need the **professional electric pump** (hospital grade) made by White River, Medela or Ameda-Egnell. Their rhythmic suctions are automatic. These heavy duty pumps are used by mothers of preemies or sick babies, and by working mothers who can leave them at the job site. These also come with the double kit for faster, more efficient pumping. These pumps are too expensive for most women to buy, but can be rented on a daily, weekly or monthly rate. Your lactation consultant or health care provider can tell you where to locate one.

Medela's Classic Pump →

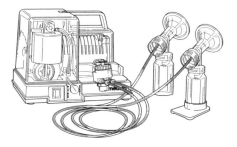

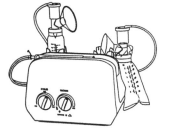

← *Ameda-Egnell's Elite Pump*

White River's rental pump →

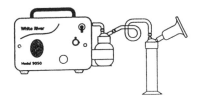

There is one pump you should **not** use - the old fashioned bicycle horn type pump. They can damage your nipples, and cannot be sterilized properly.

Choosing a breast pump to suit your needs is not easy. A La Leche League Leader or lactation consultant can help you decide which will work best for your situation. They can also tell you where to rent an electric pump.

A further word about breast pumps: Millions of mothers throughout history have breastfed without the use of breast pumps. Unless you are separated from your baby for long hours at a time, you probably won't NEED a breast pump. Sources for breast pumps are listed in the appendix.

Breast Shells

Breast shells are round plastic gadgets that fit in the bra. They are used to keep sore nipples dry and to keep sore nipples from rubbing against clothing. They are also used by women who have inverted nipples.

They work by putting a gentle pressure on the base of the nipple, which helps break down adhesions, causing the nipple to stand out. They work best when they are worn for several hours a day during the last trimester of pregnancy. However, if you need to, you can still wear them after the baby is born. Just wear them between feedings for a while. It make take several weeks to get your nipples to stand out. You can buy them from most La Leche League leaders, lactation consultants or maternity shops.

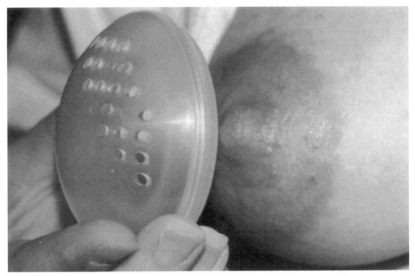

A breast shell is being used here for a sore nipple.

Nipple Shields

Nipple shields are made of soft rubber or silicone, and they fit over your nipple while nursing. They have holes in them like bottle nipples. They have been available for many years and are greatly misused. Most of the time, they do more harm than good. Nipple shields are used for sore or cracked nipples, engorgement, if the baby has trouble latching on, if the baby has a very weak suck, or for inverted or flat nipples. Most of these problems can be overcome in time, without using a nipple shield. Before using a nipple shield, you should ask your lactation consultant if you really need one.

There are several reasons why nipple shields should not be used. They may interfere with your milk supply, because your nipple will not be stimulated enough to make enough milk. Also, many babies have become "hooked" on nipple shields and will not nurse without them. And, when you use a nipple shield, the baby will not be able to empty the breast thoroughly, and you may become engorged and get a plugged duct or breast infection.

If you have been given a nipple shield because of flat nipples or a latch-on problem, and you want to get your baby off it, you might try letting him start nursing with it in place and removing it when the nipple has been drawn out enough for him to latch on.

Remember, babies with latch-on problems or very weak sucks can be trained to suck correctly with time and patience and the help of a lactation consultant. A nipple shield may seem to solve the problem temporarily, but it is very **risky.**

With that said, the fact remains that sometimes a baby will just not be able to latch on any other way other than using a nipple shield. If it comes down to a choice of formula feeding or using a nipple shield, then by all means, use the shield. Just be certain your baby gets enough breastmilk, and keep trying to get him to nurse without it. Some babies just "outgrow" the need for it after a little while. When you use a shield, make sure that the breasts are being emptied, even if it means expressing after breastfeeding.

Breast Pads

Breast pads are worn in the bra to absorb leaking milk when you have a "letdown" between feedings. There are many types of breast pads on the market and most are similar. They absorb milk and keep your nipples dry. There are disposable kinds and washable kinds. All-cotton pads seem to work better for most women. It is best to avoid the ones that are plastic lined because they hold in moisture.

Leaking sometimes happens while you are getting your milk supply established. You may leak when you are away from home and thinking of your baby, or even when you hear another baby cry. Some mothers have a lot of leaking, and some mothers never leak at all. Sometimes a mother will leak with the first baby and not leak with the second. Usually, leaking goes away in a few weeks.

If you do start to leak, and you don't have breast pads in your bra, discreetly press your arms against your breasts, and that will stop it. Leaking is not as noticeable if you are wearing a dark print blouse.

Nursing Pillows

Some mothers find nursing pillows helpful. These commercially made pillows are made of sturdy foam rubber. They wrap around the mother's waist and make it easier to hold the baby in the correct position. They are especially helpful with twins.

Be sure whatever pillows you use help keep the baby AT breast level. If they bring the baby too high, it interferes with natural breast position and may become an inadvertent cause of sore nipples.

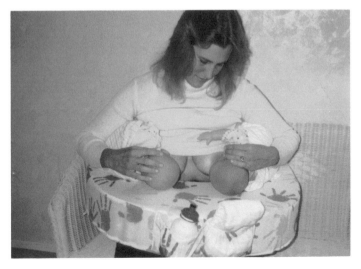

Using a Nursing Pillow with Twins

NURSING BRAS

Nursing bras are sold in many stores and catalogs. They come in all sizes, fabrics and styles. Most have "flaps" that can be unhooked to expose the nipple, but some are made of stretch fabric that can be pulled away from the nipple. Some utilize velcro, but they can be noisy when you are trying to be discreet. Nursing bras are convenient and nice to have, but you don't HAVE to have one to breastfeed. In fact, many mothers are comfortable without wearing any kind of bra. It is just a matter of preference. Mothers with large breasts usually prefer wearing a bra for support.

Under-wire bras are usually not recommended while breastfeeding, because if they don't fit properly, they may press on a milk duct and cause a plugged duct. (Some experts don't recommend under-wire bras for any women! They believe under-wires can interfere with lymphatic drainage, and may even be a factor in breast cancer.) If you feel you need an under-wire bra for more support, make sure it is fitted by a professional. Resources for nursing fashions and bras are listed in the appendix.

CARRIERS and SLINGS

It is well known that babies like to be carried. In fact, there are some babies who want (and need) to be held most of the time. If your baby *needs* to be held, then you *need* to hold him. You will not spoil your baby by carrying him. Remember, babies whose needs are met in infancy will not have as many needs as an adult.

Babies who are carried experience the world, and develop their senses faster. They don't cry as much and they learn more and thrive better. They are less bored. Carried babies are much more relaxed and secure.

A baby carrier or sling can help you carry your baby. There are front carriers, back carriers and slings. While all are convenient, many women prefer a sling because the child can sleep or nurse with the head supported. In front and back carriers, the head is not supported well and the legs are often forced apart and "dangle."

Slings are less complicated to put on and there are no belts, buckles or snaps. They are adjustable and conform to every mother's torso. And the baby's position in the sling can easily be changed. He can be placed face-out, tummy-to-tummy, lying down, or in a hip straddle position. Slings are especially useful with twins.

Some mothers believe a sling helps with sibling rivalry and jealousy. The mother is not as "tied down" to the baby and her hands are free to care for her other children.

Discreet nursing is another advantage of using a sling. Many mothers use them when they must nurse in public places.

While it is nice to own a store-bought sling, you can make your own if you can't afford one. Just take two pillowcases and carefully sew them end-to-end, making a giant loop.

You *and* your baby will love it when you wear a sling!

NURSING SUPPLEMENTER

This breastfeeding aid consists of a small bottle (worn around the neck) and a length of very small tubing which carries breastmilk or formula to the mother's nipple. The baby sucks the end of the tube and the mother's nipple at the same time. It helps to train the baby who has latch-on problems to nurse, and stimulates the breasts to produce milk at the same time.

It is also useful when a mother wants to build up her milk supply, when the baby has become nipple confused, or when an adoptive mother wants to feed at the breast. It will not necessarily help a baby, who has a poor suck, improve. It will only help him take in adequate food, and may actually reinforce poor sucking technique. Get advice from a lactation consultant. They can help you decide if you need one, and will have them available for purchase. Sources are also listed in the appendix.

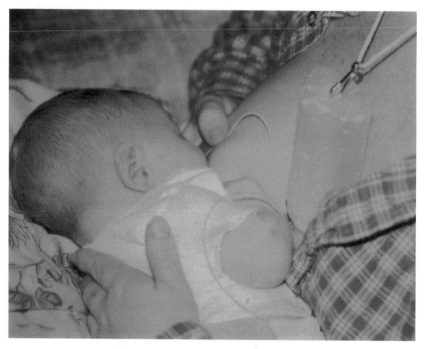

Using a nursing supplementer

Chapter Seven

Problems the Mother Might Have

---

*Nobody said breastfeeding would
always be easy. They only said it would be
worth it! I had sore nipples for a while and
a couple of breast infections. The sore nipples
were caused by poor positioning and the
breast infections were caused by "over-doing."
The first time was when we moved and
the second time was just before the holidays.
Both times I got so busy, I skipped feedings.*

Peggy

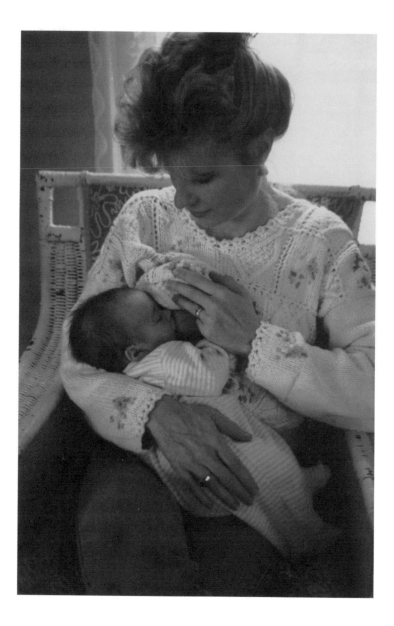

Problems the
Mother Might Have

Breastfeeding is undeniably wonderful, but sometimes there are problems that come up, both with the mother and the baby. In this chapter we will discuss problems the mother can have. While most of these problems can be an inconvenience, they can be overcome with the proper help and support of your doctor or a lactation consultant.

Cesarean Sections

Childbirth does not always go as planned. There are many mothers who end up having a Cesarean section instead of a more natural childbirth. And it can be very disappointing. But you CAN STILL breastfeed. Don't let it stop you from giving the best to your baby.

The first few days will be more difficult. But there will be people in the hospital to help you. Your nurse or lactation consultant will help you position the baby for the first few feedings, and you may find you that is more comfortable to lie down and nurse.

A Cesarean section is major surgery and it will take a while to recover completely. If you can, arrange to have help at home for the first few days. You will need to take it easy and concentrate on only two things: nursing your baby and recuperating from the surgery.

Many mothers feel that breastfeeding after a Cesarean helps "make up" for not having a more natural childbirth. (Refer to the section on positioning in Chapter 4 for more information about breastfeeding after a Cesarean.)

Most of the medications given for a Cesarean do not cause problems for the baby. Take your pain medications regularly, so you can focus on your baby instead of your pain. They will assure maximum comfort during breastfeeding, and maximum enjoyment, as well as helping you to a more rapid recovery.

Plugged Ducts

Your breasts have ducts that carry milk to the nipple pores. And, if for some reason, they are not emptied regularly, they can get "stopped up" just like a plumbing pipe.

When you have a plugged duct, you might notice a small tender spot or lump in the breast. It might happen when the baby decides to sleep through the night, or if you get busy and don't nurse as often. Sometimes a tight bra (or even a shoulder bag or seatbelt) can be pressing on a milk duct. Stress and poor nutrition can also cause plugged milk ducts. Plugged ducts are easy to correct if you catch them in time. The hardened milk that has plugged up the duct will have to be broken up and moved out. Here's how to get rid of a plugged duct:

- Take the baby to bed with you and nurse OFTEN.

- Change positions each time you nurse so that all ducts will be emptied.

- Massage the breast before nursing to help break up the hardened milk. "Combing" gently over the area (toward the nipple) with a comb may help break up the plug.

- Apply warm moist heat to the affected breast or soak it in warm water (fill up the bathroom sink with warm water, lean over it and massage) or massage in a hot shower or bath.

Early treatment for a plugged duct will help prevent getting a breast infection (mastitis).

Breast Infections/Mastitis

You will know when you have mastitis (a breast infection). You will have all the symptoms of a plugged duct PLUS headaches, aching all over, and usually a high fever. The area around the plugged duct will be red and extremely sore.

If your breast does get infected, you should use the same treatments as you did for a plugged duct, and if it doesn't clear up in a day or so, you might have to call your doctor and ask for an antibiotic. Almost all antibiotics can be taken while breastfeeding, but Keflex is often given because it does not pass through the milk to the baby.

A breast infection, treated early, will not last but a day or two. Remember to continue nursing often, because an empty breast will heal faster. And the milk from an infected breast will not harm your baby; the infection is in the breast, not your milk. Breast infections are common around holidays and other stressful times, because mothers get busy and inadvertently skip feedings. Prompt attention to breast infections is very important. Be sure to take all your medication, because if you don't, the infection may come back. Left untreated, a breast infection could turn into an abscess, which is very serious and may require surgical attention.

Sore Nipples

Some amount of tenderness at first is normal, but if the baby is held in the correct position, and is *sucking correctly*, nipples should never get to the point of blistering, cracking, or bleeding. When the baby is sucking correctly, all of the nipple will be in the baby's mouth, and there won't be any friction against it. It is friction that causes nipple damage and soreness.

Remember to get as much of the areola in the baby's mouth as possible. His body should be facing you. The chin should be touching your breast. His mouth should be open wide and both lips should be flanged (poked) out. Take your finger and pull down on your baby's chin if the bottom lip is tucked in. If he won't open wide, try opening *your* mouth wide. He may mimic you.

If your nipples do get sore, do the following:

- Make sure the baby is latching on correctly.

- Change positions at every feeding. This puts the pressure of the gums on a different spot each time (cradle hold, lying down, football hold, and across-the-lap).

- Nurse more often, but for shorter lengths of time. If you go longer between feedings, the baby will be hungrier, and may nurse too vigorously, which will make your nipples even more sore.

- Rub breastmilk on the nipples after each feeding and let them dry before putting your bra back on. Breastmilk actually helps heal sore nipples. (However, don't use breastmilk on them if you have thrush because yeast thrives on milk.)

- Don't use soap or alcohol on your nipples.

- If the pain is severe, take a mild painkiller about 30 minutes before nursing.

- Wear breast shells in your bra to keep the fabric from rubbing the nipples. See chapter 6 for more information on breast shells.

Cracked or Bleeding Nipples

If your nipples are *cracked or bleeding*, you will need to follow the same general instructions as outlined for sore nipples but you will also need to rub a small amount of **100% pure medical grade lanolin** (Lansinoh) on the nipples.

This treatment, called "moist wound healing," will relieve pain, and provide a moisture barrier that will slow the evaporation of moisture in the skin. It will allow the wound to heal much faster, without forming a scab. When scabs form on the nipple, they are usually removed when the baby nurses, which means the healing process has to start all over every time you nurse!

Medical grade, pure lanolin does not have to be removed before the baby nurses. It is available from your La Leche League leader or lactation consultant.

Occasionally, a nipple will get so damaged that the mother will have to take the baby off the breast until it heals. She will have to gently express the milk (by hand or pump) and feed the baby her expressed milk some other way (cup, medicine dropper or spoon) until the nipple heals.

Tongue-Tie

One other thing about sore nipples. Occasionally, you may be doing everything right and still have sore nipples. You may be holding the baby in the correct position, he may seem to be sucking correctly, but your nipples get sore and don't seem to improve with time. If this happens, have your pediatrician or lactation consultant check to see if your child could be **tongue-tied**. Tongue-tie means that the little piece of skin, called the frenulum, under the tongue, is tight, making it impossible for the baby to stick his tongue out far enough to suck correctly. If your baby's tongue is "heart-shaped," it is a good indication that he may be tongue-tied. Tongue-tie is fairly common and seems to run in families. It is a problem that is easily remedied by clipping the frenulum. Your doctor, dentist or nurse practitioner can probably do the clipping in a matter of seconds. It only bleeds a drop or two and baby can breastfeed immediately after. You should notice a big improvement in the way your baby sucks after his frenulum has been clipped.

Sore Nipples and Thrush

Sometimes nursing can be going along just fine for weeks or even months, when all of a sudden your nipples get sore, start itching and burning or flaking. Sometimes it may even be severe pain, deep in the breast. When this happens you most likely have a yeast infection or thrush. The technical name is *candida albicans*. Look in the baby's mouth to see if you see any white patches on his cheeks or tongue. And check to see if he has little red bumps on his bottom. If you see any of these symptoms, you can be pretty sure it is thrush. Yeast infections are usually the result of taking antibiotics, which kill off all bacteria, even the "good" kind which keeps yeast from growing. Both you and your baby have to be treated.

There are a couple of ways to treat thrush. Most doctors will prescribe nystatin drops for your baby's mouth after nursing and nystatin ointment for your nipples. Call your doctor for a prescription. The symptoms will clear up quickly, but use all the medication so it won't come back.

Another remedy is **Gentian violet**. It is an age-old

solution to the problem and is much cheaper. It can be bought at most drugstores. It is a purple liquid and a bit messy, but it almost always works. Here's how to use Gentian violet:

- Use .5% or 1% strength Gentian violet in WATER. (1% is fine and is the easiest to find. The weaker solution needs special preparation and is not as good.)

- Once a day, dip a q-tip into Gentian violet and swab the baby's mouth. Let him suck on the swab a few seconds. If this doesn't coat the entire mouth, then paint his cheeks and tongue as much as possible.

- Immediately after treating the baby, put him onto the breast, and let him nurse both breasts. If, at the end of the feeding, you have a baby with a purple mouth, and you have two purple nipples, the treatment is done for the day. But, if at the end of the feed, you don't have two purple nipples, then paint the nipple which is not.

- Repeat treatment once a day for three days. If re-infection occurs, repeat entire process once but if it occurs again, see your doctor.

- About 10 ml (2 teaspoons) is plenty for an entire treatment.

Many mothers do the treatment at bedtime so they can keep the nipples exposed and not worry about staining their clothing.

Usually there is some relief within hours and pain should be virtually gone by the third day. If it is not, Candida may not have been the problem. Seek further help.

All artificial nipples and pacifiers should be boiled daily

during the treatment or coated with Gentian violet. Toys and teething rings also must be boiled daily to keep from re-infecting your baby.

Some babies are not bothered by thrush and there is no need to treat if neither the mother nor the baby has any discomfort.

Note: It is very unusual, but some babies DO develop sores in the mouth if the Gentian violet is too strong. Discontinue at once, if this happens. The sores almost always heal within 24 hours. No special treatment is necessary.

(Gentian violet instructions adapted from a handout by Jack Newman, MD, FRCPC)

Deep Pain in the Breast

Thrush can sometimes enter the breast through a crack or fissure around the nipple. If this happens, you may feel a deep, burning or stabbing pain in the breast. It may be very uncomfortable and you will probably have to seek help from your lactation consultant or doctor. A medication named Diflucan usually helps this condition and can be taken while breastfeeding.

Breastfeeding almost never has to be stopped when you have a yeast infection on the nipples or in the breast. If it is just too painful, you can express milk with a breast pump and feed with a cup or bottle. However, a word of caution: thrush can live in frozen breastmilk, so it must never be frozen and given to the baby at a later date because the baby will be re-infected. If you have frozen breastmilk that may be infected with thrush you may still use it if it is boiled. (Some of the nutrients will be lost, however.)

Menstrual Periods

Although this is not a "problem," most new mothers worry about when they will have a period. If you are nursing *exclusively* (no solids, bottles or even pacifiers) you probably won't have menstrual periods for several months. And while there are a few women who get their period back quickly, most go much longer. It is common for women to have *lactational amenorrhea* (no periods because of breastfeeding) for 1 or 2 years if the baby is nursing often, especially at night. It depends on your hormones

Breastfeeding while you are having a period does not generally affect your milk, and is not a reason to wean. Some babies act like they don't like the taste of breastmilk, and are fussy while nursing, but return to normal once the period has passed. Your nipples and breasts might be a little tender during your period.

Can I get pregnant while nursing?

YES, YOU CAN get pregnant while breastfeeding, but it is *rare* to ovulate before you have your first menstrual period. Exclusive breastfeeding (no solids, formula, or even pacifiers) will probably protect you for the first 4 or 5 months. But, if it is important that you NOT get pregnant, use some other type of birth control.

In countries where MOST women breastfeed on demand, and they use NO birth control, the babies come about every 3-4 years.

Birth Control Pills

Birth control pills are used by many nursing mothers, but other contraceptive methods are better. The "mini" pill, (progestin only) or the Norplant are commonly used. These appear to have less effect on your milk supply and your baby's growth than the other pills. But they probably will affect both.

The "regular" birth control pill (estrogen-progestin) definitely affects your milk supply and your baby's growth. It is better to wait at least 4 to 6 months (when your baby is taking solids) before taking them.

There are other birth control options. Condoms and diaphragms are excellent choices that don't affect your milk supply or your baby's growth.

Note: Additional comments about birth control pills are found in the appendix under "Using Medications While Breastfeeding ."

Mother's Illness

Generally speaking, you should continue nursing if you get sick. Your baby probably won't catch what you have. In fact, before you even come down with any symptoms, your body will have already produced antibodies in your milk, which will help your baby fight the infection.

If you are sick enough to need medicine, make sure your doctor knows you are breastfeeding so that he can prescribe medicine that won't harm your baby. Most antibiotics can be taken while breastfeeding. Over the counter medicines are usually all right as long as you only take them once in a while. A warning: Over-use of antihistamines can dry up your milk.

The benefits of breastfeeding usually outweigh the risks of your baby getting most serious diseases. But if you do have a serious disease, discuss the benefits and risks with your doctor before making the decision to breastfeed.

See appendix A for a thorough discussion of "Using Medications While Breastfeeding."

HIV Positive and AIDS

The AIDS virus **can** be passed through breastmilk. Therefore, before **any pregnant woman at risk** makes the decision to breastfeed, she should be tested for HIV infection. You are at risk :

- if you have had unprotected sex with more than one partner,

- if your partner has had unprotected sex with someone else,

- if you have shared needles during drug use,

- if you had a blood transfusion before mid-1985,

- or if you are a hemophiliac who uses blood products.

If you have been diagnosed as being HIV + during pregnancy, taking AZT greatly reduces the chances that your baby will get HIV.

If you cannot give your baby your own breastmilk because you are HIV +, try to find a human milk bank that can provide human milk for your baby. Don't assume you must use formula with all its attendant risks.

In undeveloped countries, the advantages of breast milk outweigh the risks of developing AIDS and breastfeeding is encouraged. But in the United States, the Center for Disease Control and Prevention and the U.S. Public Health Service both have recommended that women who are HIV Positive or have AIDS should NOT breastfeed. There is still much research to be done concerning this issue.

Chapter Eight

Problems the Baby Might Have

I was so scared when they told me my baby had yellow jaundice. I thought it was something really serious. Then, I found out it was probably caused by her not nursing often enough. I went home and nursed around the clock for 3 days. When I took her back, the bilirubin level was down and she was fine. I almost quit when they told me nursing (or not nursing enough) was causing it, but now I'm glad I didn't.

Susan

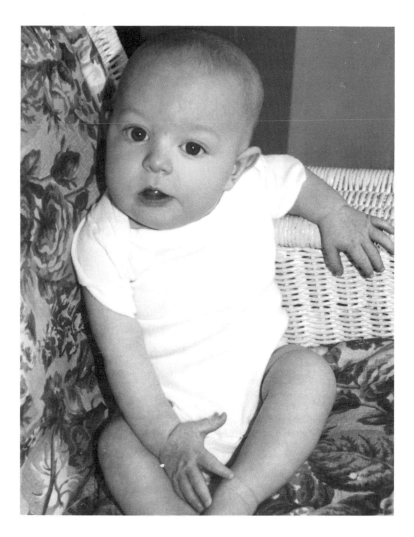

Problems the Baby Might Have

Jaundice

Although it can be frightening to hear your baby has (yellow) jaundice, it is usually nothing to worry about. More than half of all babies are jaundiced during the first week, and breastfed babies even longer. You can still breastfeed. In fact, breastfeeding frequently and effectively the first few days will usually prevent excessive jaundice.

Jaundice occurs when the baby's system can't get rid of **bilirubin**, the by-product of extra red blood cells that have built up in the womb. If your doctor suspects jaundice, he will measure the bilirubin level. If your baby is a healthy, full-term baby and the level is below 20 mg/dl and rising slowly (less than 0.5 mg/dl per hour), it is probably NOT serious. But it still must be monitored. The higher the bilirubin count, the more yellow your baby will look.

Bilirubin is passed through the stools, so the more stools your baby has, the quicker the excess bilirubin will be eliminated. Nursing often from birth will help prevent jaundice because the colostrum (which acts like a laxative) will help get rid of the meconium, the black, sticky first stools, which are loaded with bilirubin.

Some doctors, in the past, have taken jaundiced babies off the breast, and prescribed formula or water to help "flush out" bilirubin. This is not a good idea because formula can constipate babies, and make the problem even worse. And water is unnecessary because almost all bilirubin is excreted in bowel movements, not urine.

There are three types of jaundice that we will discuss. All three cause the skin and eyes to appear yellow.

Physiologic Jaundice

The first is called **physiologic** (normal) or **early onset** jaundice. It appears after the first 24 hours, peaks on the 3rd or 4th day, and gradually disappears in a week or so. **Nearly all** babies have some degree of this type of jaundice. It is self-limiting and usually requires no treatment. Early onset jaundice is sometimes called "lack of breastmilk jaundice," because early and frequent breastfeeding could have prevented it.

Pathological Jaundice

A second type of jaundice is called **pathological** jaundice. Chances are your baby does *not* have this type of jaundice. It is much more serious, and is caused by Rh or ABO blood incompatibilities between the mother and baby, infections, diseases of the liver or other rare disorders. This type of jaundice may show up within the first 24 hours and the under-lying problem must be treated promptly. Tests can quickly determine if your baby has a rare condition that would cause pathological jaundice.

"Breastmilk" Jaundice

Breastmilk jaundice (also called **late onset** jaundice) was once thought to be separate and distinct from physiologic jaundice, but experts now believe it is just the "normal extension of physiologic jaundice of the newborn."(1) Elevated bilirubin levels occur (to some degree) in about two-thirds of all breastfed infants. The levels usually peak during the second or third week and then decline progressively thereafter. These babies are growing well and developing normally.

Research has not yet identified the component in human

milk that causes this type of jaundice but one theory suggests that it is actually beneficial and may protect infants from potential illnesses.

Babies are often taken off the breast and offered formula when diagnosed as having breastmilk jaundice. This is usually unnecessary and could lead to other problems, like nipple confusion and formula allergies. Continuing to breastfeed frequently is often the best "treatment." However, on very rare occasions, when the bilirubin count becomes excessively high, it may be necessary to temporarily stop breastfeeding for one or two days. (To prevent nipple confusion, babies can be fed formula with eyedroppers, spoons, cups or bottles.)

Many doctors do prefer to treat jaundice if it reaches a certain level. The American Academy of Pediatrics recommends phototherapy when the bilirubin level reaches 20 mg/dl in a healthy newborn.(2) Phototherapy, special lights that break down bilirubin stored in the skin, is not dangerous. It may look frightening because your baby will have to wear blinders over his eyes while he is being treated. You need not discontinue breastfeeding. In fact, as mentioned before, breastfeeding often will help your baby to stool more and get rid of the excess bilirubin. Your baby can be brought to you when he needs to nurse.

Your baby may also be able to get phototherapy at home. Many lactation consultants and visiting nurses now have portable phototherapy units. They can come to your home if treatment is needed.

If your baby is only mildly jaundiced, he can be treated the old-fashioned way. Just undress him (down to his diaper) and place him near a window. Indirect sunlight will help break down bilirubin. But a word of caution: Don't ever put your baby in direct sunlight (indoors or out) because newborns burn easily.

Note: If, after you leave the hospital, your baby's skin or eyes start to look yellow, notify his pediatrician.

(1) Gartner, L., Neonatal Jaundice. *Pediatric Review* 1994b; 15(11):422-32

(2) American Academy of Pediatrics Provisional Committee for Quality Improvement and Subcommittee on Hyperbilirubinemia. Practice Paremeter: management of hyper-bilirubinemia in the healthy term newborn. *Pediatrics* 1994; 94(4):558-65

Colic

When your baby cries hard and loud for long periods of time every day, he is said to have "colic." He will act like he is in terrible pain, and nothing you do will seem to help. The screaming spells usually last 2 or 3 hours at night or late after-noon. No one knows for sure, but colic is probably caused by an immature nervous or digestive system. By the third month, most colic goes away.

Rest assured that breastfeeding is the best thing you can be doing for your colicky baby. It would probably be much worse if he were bottle fed. He is much more able to digest breast milk than formula. And nursing will help soothe him.

Your colicky baby will want to nurse often and for long periods of time, but be careful because sometimes he will over-feed, and be even more miserable. To keep him from over-feeding, try nursing every 2 hours but give him only one breast at a feeding. By feeding on one breast only, he is able to suck and be soothed, but after a few minutes, will be nursing a fairly empty breast, and won't overfeed. A pacifier may also be helpful between feedings. (Be sure to read about pacifiers in chapter five.) Your baby will need to be burped often if he has colic.

A colicky baby will need skin-to-skin contact and soft, calm handling. Sometimes a warm bath will help, and sometimes swaddling him in a blanket will help. Sometime he may need to be held and rocked, or walked. Many times bouts of colic have been helped by a patient father gently walking the baby. Mylicon drops, bought at the drugstore, help sometimes too.

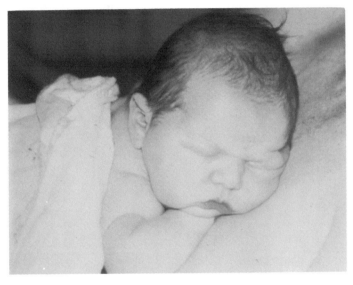

Skin-to-skin helps a colicky baby.

Sometimes colic is caused by an allergy to something in the mother's diet. Milk and dairy products are often the cause. If your baby shows signs of having colic, try eliminating all milk and dairy products for a week to 10 days to see if the colic goes away. After a few weeks, the baby may be able to handle dairy products, and you can gradually start drinking milk. It is an old wives' tale that you "have to drink milk to make milk." After all, cows don't drink milk! You can get your calcium from green leafy vegetables, or even calcium tablets.

Are you giving your baby vitamins? Sometimes they cause colic symptoms or stomach upsets. Or are *you* taking vitamin supplements? Mothers who are taking a multivitamin with iron sometimes see a drastic difference in their colicky babies when they eliminate their vitamin tablets.

Caffeine drinks can also cause colic symptoms. Cut back on these if your baby has colic.

One more thought. Some babies with colic can be helped by chiropractic adjustments. One study showed that of 316 babies with colic, 94% showed improvement in 14 days. *(Klougart, n. et al. Infantile colic and chiropractic, European Journal of Chiropractic 1985; 12 (4):281-88.)*

Premature babies

If your baby is born early, he will be much better off if he is fed your milk. It is perfectly suited to the needs of your baby, and is high in protein and other valuable nutrients. It is more easily digested than any formula, and causes less stress on baby's system. There are some hospitals that routinely give breastmilk to preemies. Some even have human breastmilk banks, which process milk from breastmilk donors.

If the baby has problems, or is very tiny, your doctor may order a special high calorie supplement especially suited for preemies. This will be given in addition to your breastmilk.

When the baby is in the hospital, you will need to pump (or hand express) the milk from your breasts and carry it to the hospital. By doing this you will be building up your milk supply as well as supplying valuable milk for the baby. A lactation consultant or specially trained nurse will teach you how to collect and transport your milk to the hospital.

Your preemie baby might have a very weak suck at first, but he will soon become stronger. The sooner you are able to nurse him, the better. Sometimes hospitals may use cup-feeding or tube feedings, or some combination of feedings until the baby is able to nurse all the time. But unfortunately, most hospitals do use bottles and nipples as the alternative, until they decide the baby can go regularly to breast. This might result in a nipple preference, or nipple confusion (as discussed in chapter 5). Sometimes if the situation is not quickly rectified, you might need to use a nursing supplementer until your baby is nursing correctly, all the time, at your breast.

Having a premature baby is stressful for the entire family. Seek comfort from friends or others who may have gone through it. Your nurse may even refer you to a support group for parents of preemies.

Having to leave your baby in the hospital will be difficult, but by giving your milk, you will feel better about it. **You will be giving your baby something no one else can.**

The day will finally come when the nurses let you breastfeed your baby. And the first few attempts may not be easy. Your baby may have become used to the bottle nipple, or he may be too weak to latch on correctly. Or he may just lick and nuzzle the breast and not know what to do. Be patient and keep trying. The lactation consultant in the special care nursery will help you. It may take time, but your preemie baby **will** learn to nurse. And in a few months, when he is growing like a weed, and nursing like a pro, you will find it hard to believe he was ever so tiny.

Illness of Baby

Even fully breastfed babies get sick occasionally, especially if there are older children in the house who bring home germs from school. But breastfed babies hardly ever get as sick as the rest of the family. Theirs is usually a mild case. No matter what illness your baby gets, it is almost always better to continue nursing. Since breastmilk is so easy to digest, it is sometimes the only food a sick baby can handle. Even when they are vomiting, they should continue to nurse. Most doctors now consider breastmilk to be a "clear liquid," and will not take the baby off the breast for gastrointestinal illnesses. Sick babies usually want to nurse more often. It is comforting to them.

Thrush

Thrush is a yeast infection in the baby's mouth. It looks like white patches on his tongue, gums and inside his cheeks. It may also show up as a diaper rash that peels, or looks like small red dots. It is often a side effect of antibiotics, that have been given to either the mother or the baby.

When a baby has thrush, it will usually spread to the mother's nipples and they will become red and very sore. When you *suddenly* get sore nipples after several weeks, or even months of breastfeeding, a yeast infection is probably the cause.

Some babies are not bothered by thrush and it may go away without any treatment. Only if the mother starts showing discomfort should treatment be started. Treatment usually involves nystatin (Mycostatin) ointment or drops. Gentian violet may also be used. (See previous chapter for Gentian violet instructions.) *Both the baby's mouth and the mother's nipples have to be treated.*

If left untreated, yeast on the nipples only gets worse. They may become inflamed, and you may have radiating pain in the breast. If ointments and drops or Gentian violet don't help, an oral medication may be prescribed.

Babies With More Serious Problems

Down syndrome: These very special babies can (and should) be nursed. In fact, breastfeeding your Down syndrome baby will be the very best thing you can do for him. He will receive love and security, as well as the valuable nutrients and antibodies from your breast. The extra effort of nursing will exercise his face and jaw muscles and will help him develop his speech skills and may prevent future orthodontic problems.

But that's not all. Babies with Down syndrome will sometimes have impaired immune systems and breastmilk is especially critical for them. Breastfeeding will ensure that they get immunities from their mother and will optimize the development of their own systems. Breastfeeding can help prevent many upper respiratory infections, including pneumonia, in these babies.

Children with Down syndrome are almost always mentally retarded to some degree. Most end up in the "mildly mentally retarded" category. Since the difference between a normal IQ score of 100 and mental retardation (technically 75 or below) is only 25 points, the extra 5-10 points he can gain by being breastfed for two years or longer may be especially critical for him.

Some babies with Down syndrome latch on and nurse without problems from the beginning. But some don't. Some have weak muscle tone and small mouths which may hinder their abilities to latch on and suck effectively.

A baby with Down syndrome may be sleepy at first and not demand to nurse very often. This is the one time you may have to nurse on a schedule. Nurse about every two hours for the first few weeks. As time goes by, and he learns to nurse more efficiently, he may go as long as 3 hours between feedings. Then again, your baby with Down syndrome may want to nurse several times an hour - he'll have his own personality, just like any other baby!

It may take lots of patience and effort, (and a little help from a lactation consultant or an experienced LLL Leader) to successfully nurse your Down syndrome child, but it will certainly be worth it. He will be a healthier child and will be the light of your life. These children bring much joy into the lives of their families.

Cleft lip and palate: Most babies born with a **cleft lip** can be breastfed. The surgical repair will be done fairly soon after birth but until then, you may have to "seal" the cleft with a finger as you nurse, or hold your baby closer to your breast. It will probably be easier if you hold him in an upright position or use the football hold.

Nursing a baby with a **cleft palate** will be more difficult and may be impossible if the cleft is extensive. Surgeons wait longer to repair cleft palates. However, some mothers have been able to nurse in the interim by using a dental appliance which seals the cleft or by using a nursing supplementer.

Nursing your baby who has a cleft lip or palate will take patience, experimenting with positions, and help from a lactation consultant. If you find you cannot breastfeed, you can still express your milk and feed it to your baby. The antibodies are especially important to these babies because they are usually more susceptible to ear and respiratory infections.

Heart conditions, Spina Bifida, Cerebral Palsy and other birth defects: Babies born with birth defects need to be breastfed, if possible. They need the greater benefit of their mother's milk and the extra closeness nursing entails. These babies are especially vulnerable to infections and the antibodies in breastmilk will help keep them well.

While it may not be easy to get these special babies to

breastfeed, it will be worth it. Ask for help from a lactation consultant and make sure your doctor knows how important breastfeeding is to you. (Sadly, you may find that many health professionals will discourage you from nursing your child born with a birth defect.)

If your baby has to remain in the hospital and isn't allowed to nurse, for whatever reason, you can still provide your milk for him. As I have mentioned elsewhere, the nurses in the special care unit will teach you how to express your milk either manually or with a pump, and will give you information about storing and transporting milk to the hospital for your baby. Many hospitals and/or insurance plans actually cover the rental of pumps when a breastfed baby must stay in the hospital.

Again, knowing that you are providing your child with something that **no one else can - your breastmilk,** will help you feel better about the situation.

Chapter Nine

Diets and Habits

---

*People told me I couldn't eat my
favorite foods if I breastfed. But I found
that I could eat anything I wanted as long
as I didn't over-do it. Once I pigged out
on really spicy Mexican food and the baby
was fussy the next day. I had to wait
a few weeks before I tried THAT again!*

Yolanda

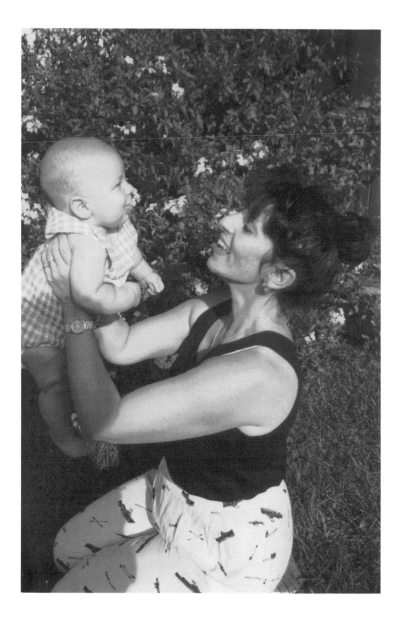

Diets and Habits

Your Diet

Many mothers think they have to give up certain foods to nurse, but this is not true. Generally speaking, you can eat anything you want to, IN MODERATION. In fact, most mothers are able to eat anything they like, without having any problems at all.

There are some babies whose digestive systems are not fully mature at birth, and spicy and gassy foods like pizza, onions, cabbage, broccoli or beans *might* make them fussy. Chocolate, strawberries, peanut butter and caffeine also may affect some newborns at first, and are things that they may have allergies to as well. Dairy products often make babies fussy.

If something seems to make your baby fussy and uncomfortable, don't eat it for a couple of weeks. Then try it again. As his digestive system matures, he can handle much more.

Ideally, you should eat a good healthy diet, just as you did during your pregnancy. Eat plenty of bread, rice, pasta and cereals and at least five servings of fruit or vegetables each day. For protein, eat lean meats, fish or poultry. You may consume dairy products as long as your baby is not sensitive to them. Learn to read labels and don't eat foods with a lot of chemical additives. You should eat about 400-500 more calories every day in the form of nutritious foods. Candy bars and soft drinks don't count! Drink plenty of water and juice (not for milk supply, but for your own optimal health.) Coffee, tea, and soft drinks with caffeine should be limited. Caffeine does pass through the milk and makes some babies restless and fussy. Try decaffeinated coffee and tea and caffeine-free soft drinks.

You will feel better if you eat a healthy diet while nursing, but *even if you don't eat right all the time, you will still make nutritious breastmilk.*

One more thing. It is not a good idea to go on any kind of reducing diet while you are breastfeeding. It won't hurt the baby, but YOUR health will suffer. And remember, as long as you don't overeat, you should be able to lose the weight you put on during pregnancy. For more information on nutritious foods, ask your doctor or other health care professional.

Alcohol, Cigarettes, and Drug Abuse

You may wonder if breastfeeding means you should give up certain things like alcohol, drug use or cigarettes. Well, the answer is yes, you should! There are certain things that are not particularly good for you and are definitely not good for your baby.

Alcohol is one of them. It is a drug, and it **does** pass through the milk to your baby. Nursing babies whose mothers drink alcoholic beverages may not gain enough weight, and their central nervous systems may be affected. Alcohol may also inhibit your "let-down" and/or decrease your milk supply.

If you **do** want to drink occasionally, make sure you do it right **after** you nurse. Drinking after nursing means the alcohol level in the milk will be low (or gone) by the next feeding. Some mothers, who anticipate a night of "partying" will express milk ahead of time to feed the baby. Then they pump and discard the milk that has alcohol in it.

Be sure there is a designated person to care for and respond to your baby's needs if you are intoxicated.

Smoking is another habit that is not good for you OR your baby. Heavy smoking has been shown to decrease the milk supply, and the level of vitamin C in the milk. And even secondhand smoke will cause your baby to have more coughs, colds, respiratory infections and may increase the risk of SIDS. If you must smoke, please don't smoke near your baby, and smoke AFTER nursing instead of just before. The nicotine levels in the milk will be lower the next feeding if you smoke after breastfeeding.

If you do smoke, and just can't seem to quit, it is very important that you breastfeed. It will help protect your baby from getting sick as often.

Recreational drugs SHOULD NOT be used while breastfeeding. Marijuana, heroin, cocaine, crack, PCP, and other illegal drugs do pass through milk and will hurt YOU and YOUR BABY. Traces of marijuana stay in your blood system (and your milk) for several weeks, and can affect your baby's development, both physically and mentally. Please don't use these drugs while breastfeeding.

See appendix "Using Medications While Breastfeeding" for a more thorough discussion on recreational drugs.

Chapter Ten

Beginning Solids and Weaning

---

*Everybody I knew had an opinion
on when I should start giving my baby
solid foods. My mother said she started me
on rice cereal when I was 2 weeks old and
thought I should do the same with my baby.
The pediatrician told me to start solids at 4
months. But my baby just wasn't ready then.
He would make awful faces and spit it out,
and he seemed perfectly satisfied with breastmilk only. I waited until he was about six
months. He was ready by then, and now (at
1 year) he eats everything I put in front of him!*

Beth

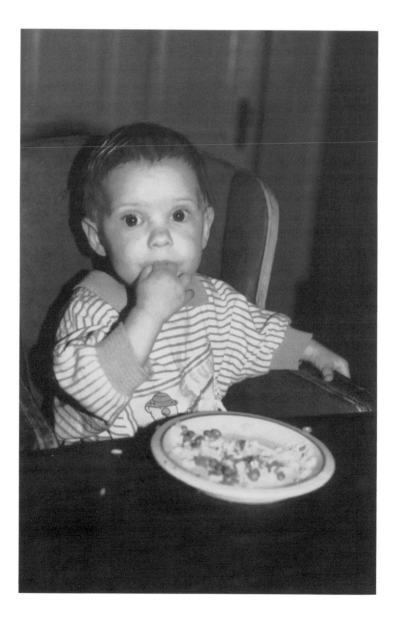

Beginning Solids
and Weaning

When to Offer Solids

When will your baby need solids? There are no clear cut answers to this question. Each baby develops at his own pace. Some babies need solids around the fourth month, and others go for almost a year before needing solid food. Six months is about average. The American Academy of Pediatricians now recommends exclusive breastfeeding for the first six months.

Your baby will let you know when he needs or wants to try solids. Around the fourth to sixth month, he may start demanding to nurse more often, and just may not seem satisfied. It could mean he is ready for solids, or it could be for some other reason, like teething. Make sure he is really ready for solids before offering them to him. There are several ways you can tell if he's ready.

Your baby may be ready for solids when:

- he starts reaching for or "asking" for YOUR food,

- he starts getting teeth,

- he can swallow solid foods without gagging,

- he can sit alone in a high chair,

- and he can hold small pieces of food in his fingers.

If he can do these things, his digestive system will probably be mature enough to handle solids.

If there is a history of food allergies in your family, you will probably want to put off solids for as long as possible. The younger the baby, the more likely he is to be allergic to certain foods.

There are other reasons for delaying solids. Babies under four months old can't digest them, and it changes the baby's intestinal flora. In other words, if your baby is doing fine on breastmilk alone, why bother with solids?

Around six months, some pediatricians get worried about anemia and recommend iron-fortified foods (or iron drops) for breastfed babies. And while it is true that breastmilk contains less iron than formula, the iron it does have is better absorbed by the baby and anemia is usually not a problem. If it will ease your mind and your doctor's, have him (or her) do a "finger stick" blood test. You will know quickly whether or not your baby needs more iron-rich foods.

There is no other food that is as good for your baby as breastmilk. As long as he is nursing you are still making milk, and he is getting those important antibodies. Even when your baby is eating solids, breastmilk should still be a major source of nutrition, well into the second year.

Note: Follow your baby's lead. If he absolutely refuses to eat solid foods, or certain foods, it may be that he just isn't ready yet for solids in general, or those foods in particular.

How do I begin giving solids?

First of all, nurse first. Breastmilk will still be the main source of nourishment for your baby. In fact, during the second six months, breastmilk should still meet three-fourths of your baby's nutritional needs. Nursing first will help maintain your milk supply.

Solids should be started slowly with just one or two feedings per day. A teaspoon or two per feeding will probably be enough to start with. Then gradually increase the amounts. If you feed your baby the same foods the rest of the family eats, he will probably show no signs of allergic reactions. Symptoms of a food allergy include: irritability and fussiness, a rash on his bottom or elsewhere, cold symptoms, ear infections or stomach upsets.

Never try to force your baby to eat. If your baby refuses a certain food one day, try again in a week or so. Forcing food could make him overweight. Many mothers don't ever spoon-feed their babies. They just wait until the baby can chew, and offer him bite-sized pieces of food which he can pick up it and eat on his own. It's easier and more natural to feed this way.

It is generally recommended that you start solids by offering certain foods in a set pattern, but this may not be necessary at all. If you start solids at six months, your baby will probably be able to handle just about anything.

If you do start earlier than 6 months, you may want to start offering rice cereal or oatmeal first. After you are sure he can handle this, offer him mashed fruits and vegetables. Most babies love bananas and enjoy picking up small pieces with their hands. Bananas are especially nutritious and easy to eat. By six or seven months, you may give him strained meat, chicken or fish. Juice may be given with a cup. When the baby is over a year old, he will probably be eating a variety of table food, but his need for breastmilk will be as great as ever. While he needs more calories and the vitamins and minerals found in table foods, he still needs your breastmilk to supply him with nutrition and immunities.

You don't have to buy commercial baby food. It is over-processed and overpriced. A small food grinder or even a fork can mash most table food to the right consistency.

Adding a little water or breastmilk to food will make it thinner. By making your own baby food, you will get the baby used to what the rest of your family eats, and save money also. Homemade foods are more nutritious than store-bought baby foods, because they don't have as much salt, sugar and non-nutritious fillers.

Ask your doctor or nutritionist for more information on what to feed your baby. Remember, for the first six months or so, breastmilk is absolutely the best thing for your baby. Nothing else even comes close.

Weaning

As soon as you start giving the baby solid foods, you are starting to wean. As the baby eats more and more solid foods, he will gradually wean from the breast.

If the baby is allowed to wean himself (baby-led weaning) he will probably wean sometime during the second year. However, since all babies are different, they can wean at different times. Some babies wean themselves during the second year, and others wean at three years or later.

It is quite common and normal if your child wants to continue nursing for a long time. In fact, it is normal to nurse for 3, or even 4, years in most parts of the world. Older children still receive the benefit of immunities as long as they nurse.

Older children who nurse get their main nourishment from solid foods, but breastmilk is still very important for them. It still provides protein, calories, fat, vitamins, minerals and antibodies. It helps keep them from getting sick, and satisfies emotional and sucking needs. Nursing is particularly helpful when your child is sick or hurt or afraid. Many toddlers, especially, benefit from nursing at nap-time and bedtime.

Studies have shown that nursing a toddler does not make him "too dependent" on the mother. In fact, satisfying his emotional needs by nursing a long time actually makes him more independent and self-reliant.

Mother-Led Weaning

When you are the one who wants to begin weaning, you must plan to do so very gradually so the baby will not feel rejected. Weaning gradually is better for you too. If you wean too quickly, you might become engorged, and get plugged ducts, leading to mastitis. If the baby is under a year old, you might need to wean him to a bottle, because he will still have strong sucking needs. Some mothers wean directly to a cup, even at this age. Other mothers wait a little longer to wean to a cup.

Begin by doing away with one feeding every few days. Start with the feeding he least enjoys. You will have to substitute formula, (or juice or snack if he is older). Mid-afternoon or mid-morning is probably a good feeding to begin with. Then after a few days, when he seems satisfied with the substitute, drop another feeding. Keep on like this until he is no longer breastfeeding. It will take several weeks to wean gently.

Your pediatrician or nutritionist can recommend which formula to feed the baby. But remember, as soon as you wean from the breast to formula, your child will begin missing out on the health benefits (and many other advantages) of breastmilk. Most doctors do not recommend cow's milk for a babies under a year old because it is so hard to digest and may cause allergies.

During the time you are trying to wean your baby, give him a lot of extra cuddling and loving. It may be especially hard for him to give up nursing at bed-time.

Note: If nursing your child for a few minutes at bedtime will get him to sleep peacefully, why not let him? There is absolutely nothing wrong with nursing your older child to sleep. You both will be happier, and he will eventually outgrow the need.

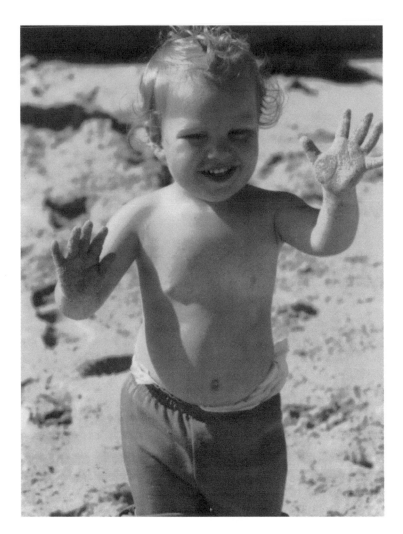

A healthy nursing toddler

Chapter Eleven

Working Outside the Home and Breastfeeding

*I never thought I could continue
breastfeeding when I went back to work.
But, I did it! It was hard at first, but
I soon got in a routine. I bought a
good little pump that I could carry
back and forth to work and I pumped
on my breaks and lunch hour. It wasn't
really that hard, once I got used to it.*

*When I picked up my baby
at the babysitter's, I would leave
the milk I had pumped that day at
her house for her to use the next day.
It was definitely worth the effort.*

Mary Ann

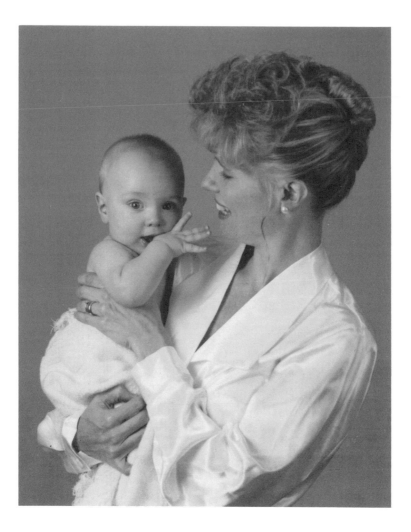

Working Outside the Home and Breastfeeding

Working outside the home and breastfeeding takes effort, but it can certainly be done. Women all over the world breastfeed while growing food for their families, fishing, herding animals, etc. And there are thousands of breastfeeding mothers who now work in offices, factories, service industries, hospitals and many other workplaces. By careful planning and with a little determination, you can do it, too.

There are many women who have no choice about working. They simply *have* to work to make ends meet. But they can still breastfeed. In fact, more and more mothers are doing it. Many believe that breastfeeding helps "make up" for the time spent away from the baby. And they are grateful for the immunities they are passing along to their babies that will help keep them from catching every little infection going around in the day care center. Breastfeeding and working takes commitment and planning, but it is well worth it.

Going back to work

It is better to wait until the baby is at least six weeks old before returning to work, and the longer you can put it off, the better. It takes about six weeks to really get your milk supply built up, and for you and your baby to really get used to breastfeeding. By then, most little problems (like sore nipples or leaking) will have cleared up. And by six weeks, your body will have recovered from childbirth.

By this time, nursing will have become much easier, and you might find it really hard to think about leaving your baby. If your finances permit, talk with your employer and see if you can take more time off. Some bosses will understand and some will not, but it won't hurt to ask.

Your Work Day

When you do go back to work, you will probably have to put your baby on a schedule. Your day will probably go like this:

- You will have to get up a little earlier, in order to have plenty of time to nurse before leaving home. Most moms have lots of milk in the mornings. Some even pump and collect the milk on one side while nursing on the other.

- Pack bottles to take to the baby-sitter. Breastmilk is best, but you can use formula if necessary. The baby-sitter will have to feed your baby about every 2-3 hours (but possibly more often if you leave breastmilk).

- Visit your baby, or have your baby brought to you on your lunch hour, if possible. If not, then pump during this time.

- Nurse the baby as soon as you can after work (at the baby sitter's if possible) and nurse on demand in the evening and during the night.

If you are working part-time, or when your baby is older and eating solids, he can drink water or juice out of a cup and eat solids when you are separated. You may not need to leave either your expressed milk or formula. And there are some babies who, rather than take a bottle, will just wait until their mothers' return. Often these babies adjust their own schedules and nurse more in the evening and during the night, and sleep more during the day at the baby-sitter's. Many mothers prefer sleeping with their babies when this situation occurs. Their sleep cycles will get in sync, and the mother will not suffer from loss of sleep.

At Work

If at all possible, you should pump your breasts at work on breaks and during your lunch hour. It will take about 10-15 minutes, depending on what type of pump you have, or how well you can hand express. You will want to save the valuable milk to give the baby-sitter for the next day so carry a small cooler, or keep it in a refrigerator at work.

If you can't pump, or do not want to pump at work, you still might have to take the pump with you for a week or so, to express milk when you get that "too full" feeling. (Just pump enough to relieve the fullness.) After you do this for a week or so, your breasts will adjust, and won't become engorged at work. You may "leak" some during the adjustment period. Wear breast pads, and see chapter three for more about leaking.

If you find that expressing milk at work is too difficult, you can leave formula for your baby. Your pediatrician can tell you what formula to use. It is always a good idea to have extra breastmilk (or formula) on hand at the baby-sitter's in case of an emergency.

Weekends

On weekends and days off you can resume nursing on demand. The breasts are remarkable. They will adjust to your routine, and you will probably have enough milk without having to use any supplements on your days off.

Planning Ahead

If you do plan to leave breastmilk for your baby, you should plan ahead. About two weeks before going back to work, start expressing so that you can store some extra breast milk. Collect milk in the mornings when you have more milk. (Some mothers find that collecting milk from one breast while the baby is nursing the other works well.) A good supply of frozen breastmilk in your freezer will give you confidence. You also need to get the baby used to taking a bottle or sipping breastmilk from a cup.

Getting the baby to take a bottle may be difficult at first. Sometimes you have to experiment with different types of nipples before you find one he will take. Putting breastmilk in the bottle will encourage him to take it. And having someone other than you give it to him will encourage him to take it.

If you don't want to use bottles, you can cup feed. Many have found cup-feeding to work very well. It just takes a little practice and even tiny babies can manage it. Use a slightly flexible cup like a plastic medicine cup or a paper cup. Place the lip of the cup on your baby's bottom lip, tilt it a bit, and let him sip the milk. Or try using a sippee cup. The newer ones have valves that keep liquid from spilling. (A word of advice: Don't try to cup-feed a newborn without the help of a nurse or lactation consultant who has been trained to cup-feed newborns. Some babies may choke.)

Collecting Milk

To collect milk, express or pump between feedings, or in the morning when you probably have an abundant supply. You do not have to collect it all at one time. Keep a bottle in the freezer, and add to it throughout the day. First, cool it off in the refrigerator, and then pour it in the bottle in the freezer. The milk will freeze in layers, and the layers might even be different colors. (What you have been eating determines what it looks like.) Shaking it well after thawing will mix it.

Collect and store the breast milk in hard plastic bottles, or disposable nursing bags. If the bags are not made especially for freezing breastmilk, double them for safety's sake. Only put two or three ounces in each bottle because your baby may not take any more than that at a feeding and any unused milk will have to be thrown out. You can always thaw out another bottle if the baby needs it. Always write the date on it and use the oldest milk first.

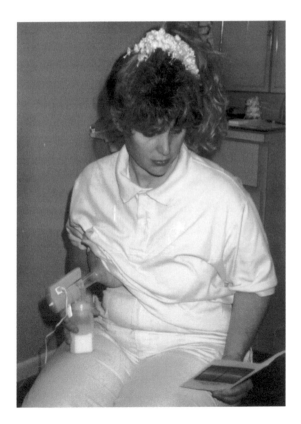

Karen, a busy chiropractor, pumps on breaks.

Storing Milk

Breastmilk can be kept in the refrigerator for about five days, and up to two weeks in the freezer section of your refrigerator. It will keep three months or longer in a deep freeze. Because it is so fresh, it will keep up to 10 hours at room temperature without spoiling.

Frozen breastmilk should be thawed out under warm running water. Never thaw it out in a microwave, because it will destroy some of the valuable nutrients, and it could cause dangerous "hot spots" that might burn the inside of your baby's mouth.

Leaving Formula

Some mothers find that they are just too tired or stressed to completely breastfeed while they are working. It **is** a great commitment, and it does take time to express breastmilk. You will feel wonderful if you can completely breastfeed your child, but you shouldn't feel guilty if you find you just can't do it. It doesn't have to be an "all or nothing" thing. ANY amount of nursing is good for your baby. Even nursing part-time will still help you give the best to your baby.

If you do plan to leave formula instead of breastmilk, make sure the baby can take it before you return to work. Some babies are allergic to cow's milk formula and have to be given soy bean formula. Your baby's doctor can tell you which formula to give.

Think Long and Hard

Most mothers don't have a choice about working; it just takes a lot of money to make ends meet these days. But if you DO have a choice about going back to work, think long and hard before you make the decision to return to work. Your baby will miss you, and you will miss your baby. No one can really take your place.

Consider all the extra expenses you will have when you work. Baby-sitters, new clothes, eating out, convenience foods, and car expenses can really add up. Add up all your expenses, and subtract it from your salary to see if it is really worth it. You might be surprised just how little money you would have left.

Can you figure out another way to manage your finances in order to stay home with your child? Perhaps you could drive your old car a while longer, or eat less fancy or convenience foods. Buy food in bulk and learn to cook "from scratch." Find a cheaper place to live. Or make do with your old clothes for a few months longer. Or, maybe your parents or in-laws could help out for a while. Many new grandparents are willing to help out financially when a grandchild's future is at stake.

Women find that with all the great technology available, it is getting easier to work out of the home. Work in the home can range from sewing or telephone soliciting to office work and professional consultations. Keeping other children is a very good way to earn extra money, too, and your child will always have playmates. Think about the talents and skills you can utilize while staying at home with your baby.

Your baby will not be a baby long, and the first few years are so important to his well-being. If you can somehow manage to stay home with your child, you will not regret it.

Chapter Twelve

Common Questions

---

*I had so many questions about
breastfeeding, I didn't know where to start.
No one seemed to have the answers. Everyone
I asked had either given up, or had not even
tried to nurse. Why isn't breastfeeding
considered normal?*

Ann

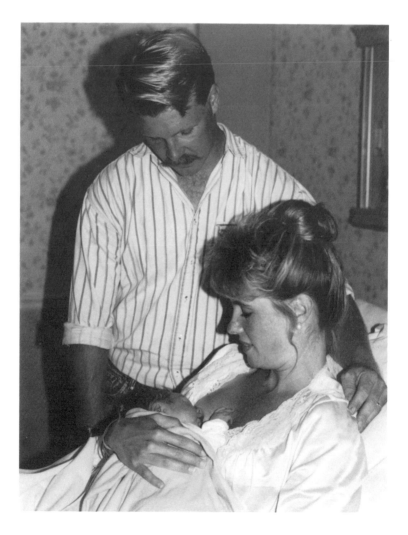

Common Questions

What exactly IS "formula"?

Formula, which is sometimes called *artificial baby milk*, is usually made from cow's milk. It has had ingredients added to it, and ingredients taken out of it, to make it more like human milk. But, there are MANY differences. Scientists will never be able to make human breastmilk. There are over 300 ingredients that have been identified in human breastmilk. Two thirds of them are NOT found in formula!

Breastmilk is alive! It is not a dead fluid from another animal. There are living cells in human milk that actually kill fungi, bacteria and viruses. Scientists will *never* be able to duplicate these cells.

Cow's milk formulas contain a different type of protein than breastmilk. Calves grow a lot faster than humans and they need more protein. These proteins are not suited for human babies. They form large curds in the stomach, and are not easily digested. Babies often suffer from digestive upsets and constipation when they are formula-fed.

Often babies are allergic to cow's milk formula, and these babies are usually given soybean formula, another inferior product. Some researchers are especially concerned about these formulas because they contain high levels of phytoestrogens, hormones that may cause developmental problems in babies. While soybean formula is easily obtained from the grocery store, it should be given *only on the advice of your physician.*

Feeding your child formula could be dangerous to his health. It is a fact that formula-fed babies get more ear infections, respiratory infections and many other serious illnesses. More formula-fed babies die from SIDS and diarrheal infections than breastfed babies. And, according to the World Health Organization, over one million babies die every year because they are not breastfed. Studies show that babies fed formula have lower IQs, and are slower to develop mentally.

Formula was "invented" in the late 1800's and was originally designed for orphaned or sick babies who could not get human milk. It was *never* meant to replace mother's milk. But large corporations saw the huge profits to be made, and through shrewd and deceptive advertising convinced the world that formula was "just as good" as human breastmilk. Many, many people (including health professionals) in the last 100 years have been deceived into thinking this. And many are still being deceived. The politics of formula feeding, money, and breastfeeding have been discussed in several books. They make excellent reading and are very thought provoking. (See appendix for suggested reading.)

A final note: You hear the argument, "I wasn't breastfed and I turned out all right." Maybe. But, maybe not. For the last fifty years or so, formula use has been a vast *uncontrolled experiment*. There are huge differences in the number of cases of heart disease, cancers and other serious conditions in countries where breastfeeding is not the norm than in countries where it is.

Formula is not "just as good" as breastmilk. It doesn't even come close! The bottom line is: **No** formulas are as good for your baby as **your** milk.

But suppose I HAVE to bottle-feed?

There are a few times when a mother has to bottle-feed. She may have a very serious chronic illness, or her child may have some serious condition that would prevent him from being able to nurse. In these cases, breastfeeding may be impossible and donor milk may be unavailable.

If your baby has to be fed formula, there are certain things that you must remember for safety's sake.

- First of all, have your pediatrician recommend which formula to buy. Choosing a formula is very serious, and it is very important that the best one is selected. All formulas are different and must be analyzed to see which one is most appropriate for your baby.

- Unless you use "ready-to-feed" (very expensive) formula, make sure the tap water you mix with the formula is safe. If you are not absolutely sure your water doesn't have harmful bacteria in it, you must boil it.

- Never use water that has been sitting in the pipes all night. This water may have high concentrations of lead or copper. Bottled water may be used safely.

- If your baby doesn't drink all his formula in one sitting, it should be thrown out. Bacteria begins to grow in formula within thirty minutes.

- When you go out, always take "ready-to-feed" so it will be sterile upon opening.

- All bottles and rubber nipples should be sterilized for the first three or four months. Sterilizing equipment can be bought at most discount stores.

- Your child will not have the protective antibodies of breastmilk, so it is a good idea to keep him away from people who may be sick and contagious.

- Always feed your child in your arms and use skin-to-skin

contact as much as possible. Don't prop up the bottle because he could choke.

- Switch arms during feedings so that your baby will have equal eye stimulation. *(Bottle-feeding instructions adapted from handout by Jan Barger, IBCLC and Linda Kutner, IBCLC. Used with permission.)*

How can I "dry up" my breasts if I don't nurse?

As soon as your baby is delivered, your breasts gear up to make milk. This happens whether you intend to breastfeed or bottle-feed. So if you are *not* planning to nurse, you may be uncomfortable for a few days.

There was once a medication on the market that was useful for drying up the breasts of women who didn't want to breastfeed. But the FDA took it off the market a few years ago after several women had strokes or other complications because of it.

Now most doctors recommend that women "bind" their breasts. This is usually done by wearing tight-fitting bras (not underwire because they can cause plugged ducts) for several days while the milk is drying up. If milk is not removed by the baby or expression, the breasts will cease making milk, and eventually the swelling will decrease. Unfortunately, some women have a few miserable days while their milk is drying up.

Some hospitals keep chilled cabbage leaves on hand for non-breastfeeding women. Placing these in the bra will help decrease swelling and also help "dry-up" milk. See chapter four for more information on using cabbage leaves.

You may also use a breast pump when your breasts get uncomfortably full. Just using it long enough to relieve the fullness will not cause the breast to make more milk.

Here's an idea! Why not put your BABY to your breast,

just long enough to relieve the fullness and uncomfortable feeling? Your breast will not be emptied, so milk production will not increase. Doing this several times a day for a couple of days will help you feel better AND your baby will get the valuable colostrum which he needs to stay well. A word of warning: Some mothers who have done this have found the experience so enjoyable, that they changed their minds and decided to nurse after all!

Can a baby be "allergic" to breastmilk?

No. A baby can be allergic to something in the mother's diet but NOT to her breastmilk. This is a common misconception and sadly, many mothers have been told this by well-meaning health professionals. A baby can be sensitive to almost anything in the mother's diet, but common ones are dairy products, peanuts or peanut butter, wheat or eggs. See chapter nine for more information on food allergies.

Can I nurse if I have small breasts?

Yes. Size has nothing to do with it. As long as you have had breast changes during pregnancy, you should be able to nurse. During pregnancy the milk glands multiply. That's why your breasts get larger. It is unfortunate that some women have been mistakenly told they couldn't nurse because their breasts weren't large enough.

Can I breastfeed if I have had breast surgery?

If you have had breast reduction surgery, it may still be possible. It depends on whether or not your ducts were cut. Most surgeons today recognize that women may want to breastfeed, and work around the ducts without cutting them.

But even if some of your ducts were severed, and you don't have a full milk supply, you can still nurse with the use of a nursing supplementer or nurse part-time and formula-feed the rest of the time.

If you have had breast implants, the answer gets more difficult. There have been many mothers who have nursed with implants, and several large studies show *no link* between implants and health problems in women due to silicone leakage. It is much more relevant as to *how* the implants were put in. Implants probably won't interfere as long as they were not inserted through the areola. Talk to your surgeon.

Will breastfeeding cause my breasts to "sag?"

No. Sagging is caused by the hormones related to pregnancy, and weight gain, not breastfeeding. Gravity, age and genetic makeup also cause sagging.

Can I breastfeed twins? How?

Yes, of course you can nurse twins. Do you think Mother Nature would send us two babies without providing for a way to feed both of them? In fact, it is much easier to nurse twins than to bottle-feed twins, because you don't have to prepare and sterilize double batches of bottles everyday. And by nursing, you will feel a special closeness with each twin individually. Since many twins are born early and have special nutritional needs, they need the extra advantage of mother's milk.

Your breasts will make enough milk for your twins. Remember, **the more the breasts are emptied, the more milk will be made.** Supplements will probably not be necessary for your twins if you are nursing them on demand.

You will want to experiment with different positions

when you nurse your twins at the same time. The football hold works well for some mothers. Just tuck a baby under each arm. Another way is to criss-cross the babies in the classic cradle position with your hands or pillows supporting them. Keep experimenting until you find the most comfortable way for YOU and your babies.

You may want to nurse the babies one at a time. This will help you bond with each baby individually. You might give each baby his own breast, or switch sides each feeding. Just make sure that each baby gets enough milk. Writing down who feeds when, and for how long may be helpful for the first few days.

Some mothers of twins have found that keeping their babies near them at night helps. If you can learn to nurse lying down, you will get more rest.

You can definitely breastfeed your twins. Throughout humankind, mothers have nursed twins, and some have even nursed triplets (and more). It may seem hard to nurse more than one baby, but bottle-feeding them will be hard, too. You will need lots of support in your decision to nurse multiples, but you can do it!

Note: This section is not intended to cover all aspects of nursing multiples. There are good books available on nursing twins, or your La Leche League Leader or lactation consultant can help you.

Can I continue to breastfeed my older child AND my baby?

Yes, you can. There are many mothers who nurse all the way through pregnancy and then go on to nurse both children. In fact, tandem nursing is normal in most parts of the world. The baby, of course, will be getting most of the breastmilk since an older child will already be eating solids. But there will definitely be enough to share. Some believe it cuts down on sibling rivalry when the older child is not pushed away (and not forced to "grow up too fast") at the arrival of a newborn.

Obviously, if you plan to tandem-nurse, you will be nursing during your pregnancy. This can sometimes be very tedious because you may have extremely sore nipples during pregnancy. (In fact, that can be one of the first symptoms.) And your milk supply will probably dwindle way, way down.

When your milk supply goes down and begins to change to colostrum your older child will probably begin to wean. Most children will nurse less and less, usually only a few minutes at bedtime. However, when the new baby comes along, and when a fresh supply of milk becomes available, some older children may become enthused and want to nurse often! Usually, this enthusiasm is short-lived, and most get tired of it soon enough.

If your older child does want to nurse often, just make sure that your infant receives what he needs first. It is especially important for the new baby to receive your colostrum. Maybe your husband or someone else can distract your older child for most feedings during those important first days.

If you are tandem nursing, make sure you are getting your proper nutrition. Eat a well-balanced diet and take vitamins if necessary. Take time to enjoy your little ones and try to get plenty of rest.

Nursing two, or even three, is possible and many mothers enjoy it. Soon both of your nurslings will grow up and leave your arms. And you will look back on the time with fondness.

Will breastfeeding "tie me down?"

You may fear that nursing will "tie you down." It won't. In fact, it may even give you more freedom. It is true that breastfed babies have to be fed more often than bottle babies, and they can't be left for long periods of time. However, after the first few weeks, and after your milk supply is well established, there is no reason why you can't leave your baby once in a while. He will learn to take a bottle from a baby-sitter.

But you will probably discover that your breastfed baby is so easy to take places that you will *want* to take him with you on outings. Many mothers don't want to leave their babies for long, and babies are welcome almost everywhere. And it is so easy to take a breastfed baby along - just grab a couple of diapers, maybe a change of clothes, and go! If you are shy about nursing in public, you can learn to nurse discreetly. See chapter 5. Or if you have to go back to work or school, chapter 11 will tell you how you can do it, and continue breastfeeding.

Whether you choose to breastfeed *or* bottle-feed, you will never again have the "freedom" you once had. But, as the days go by, and you fall hopelessly in love with your baby, your "freedom" will not seem that important any more.

What is a nursing strike?

Anytime up to the age of 2 years, but usually between the ages of 3 and 8 months, a baby may suddenly lose interest in the breast and refuse to nurse. It could be that he is teething, and it hurts his gums to nurse, or he could have an ear infection, sore throat, or cold. Sometimes there is no apparent reason. But for whatever the reason, you must try to keep up your milk supply by regular pumping. And you must continue to gently offer the breast to him. Don't ever try to force him to take your breast. It can make the problem worse.

Meanwhile, you have to find some other way of feeding the baby. You can try feeding him your expressed milk from a cup or spoon or medicine dropper. Using a bottle will make it even harder to get him back on the breast. He might quickly find that it is easier to drink from a bottle. In fact, using a bottle could have caused the nursing strike in the first place.

It may take several days for the baby to resume nursing, and during this time you will need to give him lots of skin-to-skin contact and cuddling. You can even try nursing him while he is asleep. Some babies will nurse while asleep, even when "on strike."

Don't confuse a nursing strike with weaning. Weaning occurs gradually, and strikes happen suddenly. Although this will be a very trying time, hang in there. Be patient, and keep offering the breast. Soon he will be back to normal.

Will my baby bite?

Sometimes a baby will bite when he is teething. His gums are sore and when he nurses, they hurt more. A baby might also bite if you try to nurse him when he isn't hungry, or at the end of a feeding when he has had enough. It is impossible for a baby to bite and nurse at the same time because the baby's tongue is between the bottom teeth (or the gum) and your nipple, when he is nursing. Only when he has stopped nursing, will he be able to clamp down. And when a baby bites, it hurts, even if he doesn't have teeth yet.

If your baby has started biting, watch him carefully while nursing. When he stops sucking or swallowing, break the suction and take him off the breast *before* he bites.

If he does bite, gently take him off the breast and firmly say "no." After two or three times, most babies will get the message that they must not bite. If he clamps down with his teeth, and won't let go, (ouch!), bring his nose in closer to the breast, so that he will have to open his mouth to breathe. (This is not as cruel as it may sound. It only takes a second.)

Contrary to what you may hear, you DO NOT have to wean the baby when he gets teeth.

What about Dad? And sex??

A new baby in the house affects everyone, especially the father. He will have many adjustments to make. The baby will be the center of your life for a while, and your husband may feel a little left out. He may even be a little jealous of the time you spend with the baby. But there are ways that you can make him feel a part of the breastfeeding experience.

Share the breastfeeding time with him by having him sit with you while you are nursing. Talk to him about the baby, find out how he thinks the baby is getting along. Or talk to him about other things that interest him. He will appreciate your efforts to include him. Many fathers feel very protective and MANLY watching you doing something so WOMANLY.

If you think you should bottle-feed so your husband can share equally in the feeding duties, think again. Most dads help out with one or two bottles a day for the first week or so, and seldom, if ever, do it again. This sounds harsh, but ask around; it's true. You and your baby shouldn't have to miss out on all the joys and advantages of breastfeeding just so dad can give a few bottles in the early days of your child's life!

There are other ways the father can share in the care of the baby. He can help bathe him, change his diaper, play with him, take him for walks, and even go along on trips to the doctor. Fathers can also help with feedings by getting and changing the baby beforehand, and/or by bringing mom a drink or snack while she is breastfeeding. He can also help adjust pillows, and give back rubs or foot rubs while mom is feeding the baby.

Fathers are especially helpful when it comes to calming a crying baby. Many a father has been able to quiet a colicky baby, (when nothing else worked) by putting him on his strong shoulder and "walking" him.

It helps if the father knows all about breastfeeding and is aware of the many benefits. Give him this book to read, or at least convince him to read the first chapter. The father should offer encouragement and support and remember that breastfeeding should be a top priority for a while.

A new baby in the family is very stressful, whether it is breastfed *or* bottle-fed. And relationships can get rocky. Your sex life may even suffer. After spending all day caring for your infant, sex may be the last thing on your mind. You may feel "all touched out" at the end of the day. Recognize what is happening and take time out for each other. Plan your "romancing" around baby's naps. If sex is painful, or you have vaginal dryness, call your doctor. It is related to hormonal changes and your doctor can tell you what to do.

Remember, as babies get older, they get a lot less demanding of you, and you will have more time for your husband.

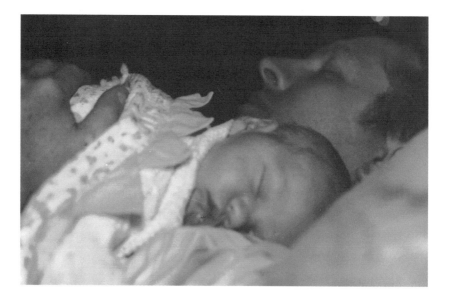

Daddies need time with baby, too.

Can I breastfeed my adopted baby?

Absolutely. There are many mothers who have nursed adopted babies. Breastfeeding is a special gift an adoptive mother can give her baby. Bonding will be enhanced and the infant will receive valuable nutrients and antibodies found in breastmilk. The key to successfully nursing an adopted child is to realize that the amount of milk you produce is *not* an indication of how well you are succeeding. Even if you are only able to provide a small part of the milk your baby needs, you are still providing him with that extra love and attention that he needs.

Usually if an adoptive mother begins pumping her breasts a couple of months before the baby's arrival, she will have stimulated them enough to make milk. (A hospital-grade, double pump setup is best.) And certain medications are sometimes prescribed to speed the process. (Milk production is a side-effect of an anti-nausea medication, Reglan, and is commonly prescribed for building up milk supplies.)

Success depends on the baby also. Many times babies are already dependent on a rubber nipple when the adoptive parents get them. While there are certain "tricks" to getting a baby to nurse, if he absolutely refuses the breast, there is not much a mother can do.

Skin to skin contact, letting the baby nuzzle the breast often, and attempting to nurse while your baby is asleep might help. "Water rebirthing" is another idea. Lie back in the bathtub with your baby on your abdomen and encourage him to crawl toward your breasts. Many mothers who have tried water rebirthing say their babies latched on then, when nothing else had worked.

Again, it is important to say that mothers who have never given birth or lactated will probably not be able to produce enough milk to completely sustain their babies. Most have to supplement with formula or with donated breastmilk. But it doesn't really matter *how much* actual breastmilk the mother provides. The very act of nurturing the baby at the breast is what's important, and will benefit the mother and the baby.

Adoptive mothers can also use nursing supplementers (see chapter 6) which will transfer supplements to the baby while stimulating the breasts to make milk.

There are many LLL Leaders and lactation consultants who are experienced in helping adoptive mothers. Contact them for more help.

Can I relactate if I need to?

Yes, women who have given birth, but for one reason or another did not breastfeed, can still relactate, even after several months. Frequent stimulation to the breasts by the baby or by pumping will bring the milk back. A lactation consultant can help you if you want to relactate. There have been mothers who have had to relactate when they found their babies were allergic to all types of formulas. And some have had to relactate in emergency situations (natural disasters, wars) when they couldn't get formula.

How do I hand express my milk?

The very best way to collect breastmilk for your baby is to "hand express" it. It stimulates the nipple more than a breast pump, and it helps maintain your milk supply better. With practice, some women become very efficient at hand expression. Manual expression helps a mother to establish, increase or maintain her milk supply when her baby cannot breastfeed.

Milk is produced in milk producing cells (alveoli). A

portion of the milk continuously comes down the ducts and collects in the milk reservoirs (sinuses).When the milk-producing cells are stimulated, they expel additional milk into the duct system. This is called the milk ejection reflex or let-down.

Chele Marmet, IBCLC, of the Lactation Institute and Breastfeeding Clinic in Encino, California, has developed the most effective method of manual expression. Follow her instructions carefully for success.

The Marmet Technique of Manual Expression

Expressing the Milk
Draining the Milk Reservoirs

1. POSITION the thumb and first two fingers about 1 to 1 ½ inches behind the nipple.

- Use this measurement, which is not necessarily the outer edge of the areola, as a guide. The areola varies in size from one woman to another.

- Place your thumb pad above the nipple and your finger pads below the nipple, forming the letter C with the hand as shown.

- Note that your fingers are positioned so that the milk reservoirs lie beneath them.

- Avoid cupping the breast.

2. PUSH straight into the chest wall.

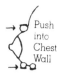

- Avoid spreading the fingers apart.
- For large breasts, first lift and then push into chest wall.

3. ROLL thumb and fingers forward as if making thumb and fingerprints at the same time.

- The rolling motion of the thumb and fingers compresses and empties the milk reservoirs without hurting sensitive breast tissue
- Note the moving position of the thumbnail and fingernails in the illustration.

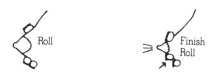

4. REPEAT RHYTHMICALLY to drain the reservoirs.

- Position, push, roll; position, push, roll...

5. ROTATE the thumb and finger position to milk the other reservoirs. Use both hands on each breast. These pictures show hand positions on the RIGHT breast.

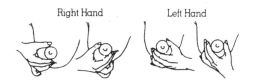

AVOID THESE MOTIONS

- Avoid squeezing the breast. This can cause bruising.

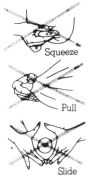

- Avoid pulling out the nipple and breast. This can cause tissue damage.

- Avoid sliding on the breast. This can cause skin burns.

Assisting the Milk Ejection Reflex
Stimulating the Flow of Milk

1. MASSAGE the milk producing cells and ducts.

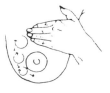

- Start at the top of the breast. Press firmly into the chest wall. Move fingers in a circular motion on one spot on the skin.
- After a few seconds, move the fingers to the next area on the breast.
- Spiral around the breast toward the areola using this massage.
- The motion is similar to that used in a breast examination.

Massage

2. STROKE the breast area from the top of the breast to the nipple with a tickle-like stroke.

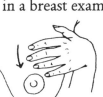

Stroke

- Continue this stroking motion from the chest wall to the nipple around the whole breast.
- This will help with relaxtion and will help stimulate the milk ejection reflex.

3. SHAKE the breast while leaning forward so that gravity will help the milk eject.

Shake

Procedure

This procedure should be followed by mothers who are expressing in place of a full feeding and those who need to establish, increase or maintain their milk supply when they baby cannot breastfeed.

• Express each breast until the flow of milk slows down.
• Assist the milk ejection reflex, (massage, stroke, shake) on both breasts. This can be done simultaneously.
• Repeat the whole process of expressing each breast and assisting the milk ejection reflex once or twice more. The flow of milk usually slows down sooner the second and third time as the reservoirs are drained.

Timing

The *entire procedure* should take approximately 20-30 minutes.
• Express each breast 5-7 minutes
• Massage, stroke, shake.
• Express each breast 3-5 minutes.
• Massage, stroke, shake.
• Express each breast 2-3 minutes.

Note: If the milk supply is established, use the times given only as a guide. Watch the flow of milk and change breasts when the flow gets small.

Note: If little or no milk is present yet, follow those suggested times closely.

Used with permission Chele Marmet, 1998.

Chapter Thirteen

Where to Turn for Help

---

*I don't know what I would have
done if I hadn't had my WIC breastfeeding
counselor to help me. I was already on
WIC and they were over-joyed that I
wanted to nurse. I had so many questions
and also some problems the first few days.
I didn't even know the WIC counselor
was a certified lactation consultant until
I had those problems. She made me feel
important and really helped me
and kept me going for almost a year.*
                    Renee

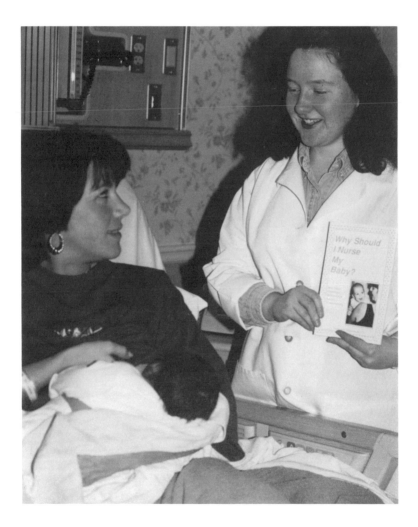

Where to Turn for Help

Lactation Consultants

A lactation consultant is a professional health worker who works with breastfeeding mothers and babies. She (or he) is trained to help the mother manage lactation and to help her become self sufficient in breastfeeding.

Lactation consultants work in hospitals, public health clinics, doctors offices and private practices. Some teach breastfeeding classes and offer telephone counseling.

Some certified lactation consultants are board certified by the International Board of Lactation Consultant Examiners (IBLCE). This organization, formed in 1985, administers a yearly examination in several countries. Lactation consultants who are board certified by the IBLCE are considered to be the best qualified. They are allowed to use the initials IBCLC (International Board Certified Lactation Consultant)behind their names.

All are professional health care providers who are experienced in lactation consultation, graduates of lactation consultation educational programs, and are breastfeeding counselors who have extensive hands-on experience in lactation consultation.

Lactation consultants are the newest members of the health care team. They work with doctors, nurses and other health care professionals who work with breastfeeding mothers. For more information on lactation consultants, contact:

International Lactation Consultant Association
4101 Lake Boone Trail, Suite 201
Raleigh NC 27607
919-787-5181   fax 919-787-4916

La Leche League

La Leche League International is recognized as the world's authority on breastfeeding. It was started in 1956 by a group of breastfeeding mothers and has grown to become a well known worldwide organization of over 3500 groups.

Their mission is "to help mothers worldwide to breastfeed through education, encouragement, and mother-to-mother support, and to promote a better understanding of breastfeeding as an important element in the healthy development of the baby and mother."

Mothers and their nursing babies meet once a month at LLL meetings to discuss such things as the advantages of breastfeeding, the baby's arrival, overcoming difficulties and nutrition and weaning. These informal meetings give mothers a chance to discuss their feelings and any problems they might have with breastfeeding. They leave the meetings grateful for the experience of finding other mothers much like themselves. Many lasting friendships begin at La Leche League meetings.

An experienced and accredited Leader "leads" the meeting and helps answer questions. Most groups have large lending libraries with much parenting information. LLL Leaders also do free phone counseling and are happy to share their breastfeeding experience with others. They do not give medical advice. For more serious problems they will refer you to a professional advisory board made up of doctors and other professionals who deal with nursing mothers.

To find out if there is a group near you or if you wish more information contact:

La Leche League International
P. O. Box 4079
Schaumburg Il 60168 USA
(708) 519-7730
For breastfeeding help: **1-800 LALECHE**
Internet address: http://www.prairienet.org/llli/homepage.html

Nursing Mothers Counsel, Inc.

Nursing Mothers Counsel, Inc. has served breastfeeding mothers since 1955. The volunteer force of nearly 400 members is dedicated to helping women enjoy a happy, healthy and practical feeding relationship with their babies.

There are chapters in various cities in California as well as Colorado, and Indiana. You may call them for a local contact number.

A packet of breastfeeding information covering the "how-to's" of breastfeeding, positioning the baby, combining working and breastfeeding and how to store breast milk is available by writing to the following address.

Nursing Mothers Counsel, Inc.
P. O. Box 50063
Palo Alto CA 94303
(415) 599-3669

WIC

The Supplemental Nutrition Program for WOMEN, INFANTS, and CHILDREN (WIC) is a U.S. federal government food program for pregnant and breastfeeding women, their infants, and their children up to age 5 years. Since the goal of WIC is to have healthy mothers and children they provide some of the foods needed for good health. Special WIC vouchers or coupons for foods such as milk, eggs, cereal, cheese, juices, beans, and peanut butter are given to the mother and are redeemed at the grocery store. Vouchers for artificial baby milk are given to bottle feeders. Breastfeeding moms get MORE food for themselves and they get EXTRA foods like tuna and fresh carrots.

To qualify, you and your baby must need extra food to be healthy, and you must meet certain income standards. You also have to live in an area that has a WIC clinic, and you have to go there for regular appointments.

WIC employees know how important breastfeeding is to growing babies and they are very supportive of it. Some WIC offices have special Breastfeeding Peer Counselors. They are other mothers who have successfully breastfed and are trained to help you. And some WIC offices have professional Lactation Consultants to help you.

If you are not already on WIC, call your local Public Health Unit for information. They can tell you where and how to apply.

Don't be afraid to ask WIC for help if you have problems breastfeeding. They want you to enjoy your baby and keep him healthy by breastfeeding a long time.

Help Outside the USA

La Leche League is an international organization and has contacts all over the world. The staff at headquarters in Schaumburg, Illinois will gladly give you the name and address of a contact person outside the United States.
Telephone: (708) 519-7730

Australian Lactation Consultant's Association is a nationally respected, professional association whose goal is the protection, promotion and support of breastfeeding as the optimal choice for both infant and maternal health. Members must be board certified by the International Board of Lactation Consultant Examiners. They may be contacted at the following address:

ALCA, INC.
P. O. Box 192
Mawson ACT 2507
Tel/fax (02) 6290 1920

Nursing Mothers Association of Australia is an organization of people whose primary goal is to protect and promote breastfeeding. Members include nursing mothers, doctors, midwives, lactation consultants and other health professionals. Founded in 1964, NMAA is known to be a source of accurate information about breastfeeding management and research. Their address:

Nursing Mothers' Association Australia
5 Glendale St.
P. O. Box 231
Nunawading 3131 Victoria, Australia
613 9877-5011

The National Childbirth Trust helps breastfeeding mothers in the United Kingdom. They offer "information and support in pregnancy, childbirth and early parenthood, and aim to enable every parent to make informed choices. They work toward ensuring that its services, activities and membership are fully accessible to everyone." Their address:

National Childbirth Trust
Alexandra House
Oldham Terrace
Acton London W3 6 NH
0181 992 8637

Appendix

Using Medications In Breastfeeding Mothers
by Thomas Hale, R.Ph., Ph.D.

The number of women in the United States who breastfeed their infants today has increased to 58% compared to only 22% in 1972. An incredible array of new evidence clearly shows that infants who are breastfed are far healthier. Significant decreases in the incidence of inner ear infections, Sudden Infant Death Syndrome, viral diarrhea, and a reduced morbidity with respiratory syncytial virus (RSV) infections provide indisputable evidence that breastfeeding is the preferred method for nourishing an infant. At the same time we also know that a great many women will be exposed to medications (perhaps 99%) during their breastfeeding experience. It has been an ongoing tendency in the past for most physicians to advise the mother to discontinue breastfeeding her infant while she is undergoing medical treatment. While to many physicians this sounds easy, it can be traumatic and is unnecessary for most lactating women. Consequently, there has been a new trend in the last few years to evaluate medication usage in lactating women so that breastfeeding can be continued without the safety of mom or infant being threatened. Each case requires a close evaluation of the mother's condition plus significant knowledge of the medication itself along with other factors such as the age of the infant. Hence, this review is a short primer on how to appropriately evaluate each situation so that both mother and child are safeguarded.

The Effects of Drugs on Lactation

While considering drugs and their penetration into reastmilk, we seem to forget that some drugs can change the lactation process itself. Although the number is very small, several drugs have been found to produce profound decreases in breastmilk. The most common of these are the oral contraceptives, particularly those that contain estrogen, which is the component that reduces the production of milk. If birth control pills are started too soon after lactation has begun, a reduction in the mother's milk supply occurs. This can have a direct effect on the baby's weight gain.

Two factors are important in evaluating birth control medications: First, the progestin-only mini pill is preferred as it has not been shown to alter breastmilk production in most women. Secondly, if a combination oral contraceptive is used (one which contains both estrogen and progestin), the mini or low dose preparations should only be used and ideally started after about six weeks into lactation. If started before that time, they can cause a reduction in milk supply. Depo-Provera has become increasingly popular for breastfeeding mothers since it does not apparently reduce the milk supply. Although this may vary from mother to mother, using Depo-Provera at four to six weeks is generally safe for infants and breastfeeding mothers. A question often asked regards the concern about whether estrogen and progestin in these products can feminize male infants. Thus far, no study on these hormones has documented any developmental changes in male breastfed infants.

Drug Penetration into Breastmilk

It is safe to say that all drugs penetrate into milk; however, the absolute amount present in milk is often only 1% or less of the mother's dosage. The amount the infant receives is often extremely small. Although this can vary between drugs, it is important to understand that all drugs will enter breastmilk. It is up to the mother and physician to decide whether the risk to the infant is minor, as is often the case, or major. Drugs penetrate into milk largely as a function of their individual chemistry and there are a number of tools which can be used to help reduce the exposure of the infant. These will be described later. Many people think that milk is a filtered product from the blood. This is simply not the case. It is created under a very tight and well controlled manner by the alveolar epithelial cells in the breast. As such, most drugs are presented to the breast tissue from the mother's blood vessels (capillaries). During the first week or so postpartum, the breast tissue is not well organized and it is possible for drugs to slip into milk rather easily. During the first two weeks postpartum, medications may reach their highest concentration in milk, although the absolute amount transferred is still low. Caution should be used during this time. In addition, infants' gastrointestinal tracts are not yet well developed and may absorb drugs in higher concentrations than would occur several weeks to a month later. Mothers should be most careful concerning drug use and breastfeeding during the first month of their infant's life. This is especially true for premature infants. After that time, infants rapidly develop the ability to metabolize drugs and are somewhat less susceptible to medications. However, most of the drugs used early postpartum (pain relievers, antibiotics, and certain antihypertensives) are generally safe for your baby.

Drugs enter and exit milk as a function of the mother's blood levels. As the level of drug in the mother's plasma increases, the amount that enters the milk also increases. As the mother's blood levels begin to drop, many drugs exit from the milk back into the mother's blood stream. This is important, because, if possible, a mother would not want to breastfeed when the drug was reaching its highest level in her bloodstream. She would need to wait an hour or so when the drug begins to drop, therefore exposing her infant to smaller levels of drug. We call this "breastfeeding away from the peak," and with drugs that are short-acting, it's a very handy technique to reduce an infant's exposure. This technique works great for penicillins, aspirin, acetaminophen and hundreds of short half-life drugs. Unfortunately, it won't work for long-acting drugs. In order to "breastfeed away from the peak," the medication needs to be taken immediately after nursing, then hopefully at the next breastfeeding time, say in 2-4 hours, the plasma level of drug will be much lower.

Typical Medications and Their Safety

Antibiotics: Certainly one of the most commonly used family of drugs are the antibiotics, particularly during this time period. Fortunately, this family of drugs almost uniformly produce only very small levels in breastmilk. The most significant complication is a change in the infant's GI tract flora, which can cause diarrhea and colitis. In some infants, this could lead to thrush or Candida overgrowth. Infants are generally colonized with Candida anyway and antibiotics may make it develop more rapidly. Although diarrhea and Candida are generally not that serious, bloody diarrhea is a reason for concern and the mother should report this to her physician.

Penicillins and Cephalosporins: The penicillin and cephalosporin antibiotics fortunately produce breastmilk levels generally far less than 1% of the maternal dose, often less than 0.1%. In general, infants can continue to breastfeed while mom is being treated with most penicillins and cephalosporin drugs. The only major complication is either a skin or allergic rash in the infant, or a change in the bacterial flora of the infant's gut. It is possible to see diarrhea in some infants but it is extremely rare.

Erythromycin: The erythromycins are a safe family of drugs for a breastfeeding mother. New studies have shown that the levels that enter milk are really quite small. A newer popular member of this family, azithromycin (Zithromax), has recently been found to produce exceptionally small levels in milk. In addition, several members of this group now have pediatric formulations which are used in pediatric patients routinely.

Sulfonamides: Although the sulfonamides are considered a very safe group, their use in the last trimester of pregnancy, or the first month of an infant's life, is discouraged because they can increase jaundice in infants. Generally after 14-30 days of life, most infants can be treated with sulfonamides. The breastmilk levels of sulfonamides are really quite small and thus far have produced no problems in breastfeeding infants; however, if possible, it is generally better to use other antibiotics at least until the infant is a month or older. Some of the newer products that contain trimethoprim such as Septra and Bactrim have been used in pediatric patients for years, thus far with few side effects, but it is better to wait until after 30 days of life. This is particularly so for premature infants.

Fluoroquinolone: The fluoroquinolone antibiotics, which consist of Cipro, Floxin, and Noroxin, are primarily used for urinary tract infections, but also for pneumonia and other gram negative infections. This group should be used with some caution. These drugs have been reported to cause diarrhea and colitis in some infants, but they are not absolutely contraindicated. One member, Norfloxacin, appears to produce the smallest milk levels of this family, and would be preferred.

Metronidazole (Flagyl): This antibiotic is used both for anaerobic bacterial infections but also for trichomonal vaginal infections. For bacterial infections, it is given as 3 tablets daily for 7 days. For trichomonas, it can either be given three times daily, or as a one-time dose of 2 gms (8 tablets). If the one-time dose is prescribed, a mother should probably stop breastfeeding and pump for at least 12 hours or perhaps up to 24 hours. Blood levels of metronidazole drop to only 20% of the peak in about 12 hours, and it is probably safe to breastfeed after 12 hours.

There is some controversy as to whether a mother should breastfeed when metronidazole is administered for up to 10 days. Thus far many do, and there have been no reported side effects yet. A new intravaginal gel has been developed. The absorption of metronidazole from the vagina is minimal and poses no problem to a breastfeeding infant.

Aminoglycosides (Gentamicin): These drugs are generally only used in hospitals by intravenous drip. Further, they are so poorly absorbed from the gut, even that of an infant, that they pose no danger to the breastfeeding infant. But observe for changes in GI flora and diarrhea.

Pain Medications

Opiates: The opiate analgesics are used for major pain. They consist of morphine, demerol, fentanyl and a number of others. In general, morphine levels in milk are quite low, and oral absorption is rather poor, so they pose little risk to a breastfed infant. Demerol, on the other hand, has a long half-life metabolite that has caused significant sedation and developmental delays in infants. It should not be used in delivery or postpartum.

Fentanyl breastmilk levels are low and it has a rather

short half-life, so it poses little risk. Codeine and its cousin, Vicodin, have been extensively used in breastfeeding mothers without undue problems. Codeine levels in milk are quite low. Again, attempt to breastfeed away from the peak level of the drug by waiting several hours or more to breastfeed.

Nonsteroidal analgesics: This is a huge family of drugs with such members as Naprosyn, Alieve, Ibuprofen, Advil, and dozens of others. In general, the penetration of these drugs in breastmilk is rather low and they are probably safe if used briefly. Of this family, Ibuprofen is uniquely preferred because it is safe to use in young infants and its penetration into breastmilk is exceptionally low.

Acetaminophen: This medication enters milk only poorly, and the levels are very low. It is safe to use in moderate to low doses. Long-term high doses should be avoided.

Aspirin: Aspirin is considered safe to use because its levels in breastmilk are low; however, we now believe that aspirin is associated with a severe syndrome in children called Reyes' syndrome. It is possible, although not likely, that a mother ingesting aspirin when her infant is ill with a viral illness could induce this syndrome. With all the safe analgesics currently on the market, it is probably best not to use aspirin routinely, if at all, while breastfeeding.

Anticonvulsants: It is not uncommon for breastfeeding mothers to require anticonvulsant medications for treating epilepsy. We have a great deal of experience with this family of drugs and in general most are considered safe to use in lactating mothers. All of these products enter milk to some degree, and will in some cases produce low but measurable levels in breastfeeding infants. If concerned about the infant, a physician can measure the amount of drug present in the infant's plasma. It is really quite easy to do, and will provide the clinical information both mother and physician need. The classic side effects of this family of drugs are primarily sedation and slowed breathing. Even though these are extremely uncommon, infants should be observed closely for weakness, sedation, and slow respiration.

Cold remedies: Cold and cough remedies fall into the category of drugs of questionable efficacy. The main question a mother should ask is, "Is this drug really necessary, and can I do without it?" If your answer is yes, then it is best not to use these products. We know little about breastmilk levels of antihistamines and decongestants other than they have been reported to produce sedation in some infants, and agitation and hallucinations in others. A little codeine (15 mg) as a cough syrup is probably fine, but otherwise, this group is of little use and should be avoided. Nasal sprays produce only small plasma levels and are probably safe to use but in general are not recommended.

High Blood Pressure Medications: Although these medications are infrequently used, there are a number of instances where they are needed. Some of these preparations can pass into milk in high enough levels to produce side effects in breast-feeding infants, particularly since they are used for long periods. Several members of the beta blocker family have produced significant problems in infants. Propranolol is a preferred member of this group. If the beta blocker family is used, observe the infant for decreased breathing, low blood sugar, and weakness. In the calcium channel family, nifedipine produces rather low levels and is probably preferred. We have little data on this family, but thus far nifedipine appears to be a preferred product. The ACE inhibitor family should be used cautiously, as pediatric patients are extremely sensitive to this group, but there are several in this family that attain low milk levels.Overall, the main problems associated with all antihypertensives are sedation, slow heart rate, and low blood pressure. If these are noted in the infant, the mother should notify her physician. The type or dose of the medication should be changed, or breastfeeding should be stopped if no other alternative exists.

Dental Medications: The primary medications used by dentists include local anesthetics, penicillin antibiotics, and opiate analgesics such as codeine, or occasionally Demerol. As mentioned before, Demerol should not be used, but single doses such as during surgery probably pose little problem. Codeine or Vicodan should be suggested as alternative analgesics. The local anesthetic, lidocaine, produces only minimal breastmilk levels, generally far less than 40% of the mother's plasma level. Only about 15% of Lidocaine is absorbed orally, so it is extremely unlikely it will produce any side effects in a breastfeeding infant. But just to be safe, the mother could pump and dump for up to 4-6 hours after receiving the medication, and most would already be eliminated from her plasma, although this is probably not necessary.

Vaccines: Almost without exception, most vaccines are safe to use. Vaccines consist either of killed virus or one that is weakened or attenuated. All killed vaccines are safe to use in breastfeeding mothers. The only live attenuated vaccine that should be used with caution is the oral polio vaccine. This is not because it is unsafe for the infant, but because we believe that it may reduce the infant's antibody production at later exposures.

Radiologic or Diagnostic Tests: A number of drugs are used as contrast agents during CAT or MRI scans. In addition, other radiologic procedures may use radioactive compounds. If a radioactive compound is used, the mother should interrupt breastfeeding until it is completely decayed, which generally takes 5 half-lives. Ask the physician how long the half-life is, and multiply it by 5. If radioactive Iodine-131 or Iodine-125 is used, most mothers should permanently stop breastfeeding. These two isotopes have long half-lives and worse, can concentrate in and destroy the infant's thyroid gland. For thyroid scanning, suggest that the radiologist use Iodine-123, a short half-life product. However, most CAT and MRI scans use radio contrast agents (non-radioactive) that are rapidly cleared from the body, and even if they were to enter milk, they are not absorbed orally by the infant. For these preparations, mothers should interrupt breastfeeding for a few hours at most.

Drugs of Abuse: Drugs of abuse are used for their powerful effect on the brain. Drugs that readily enter the brain compartment, readily enter breastmilk as well. All powerful brain-altering drugs should be avoided by breastfeeding mothers at all times. Cocaine, marijuana, phencyclidine (PCP) readily enter milk in high levels. Urine tests of the infant will be positive for PCP or marijuana for up to a month or longer. Cocaine will be present in an infant's urine for 2-3 weeks. Do not use these products and continue to breastfeed. An infant can inhale enough crack cocaine while it is being smoked to become agitated, colicky, and test positive in urine screens, so do not smoke cocaine around your infant.

Antidepressants: The use of antidepressants in postpartum breastfeeding mothers is the most controversial subject in the breastfeeding literature. All antidepressants are secreted into human milk to some degree. The tricyclic family of antidepressants have been used for many years and we have a great deal of experience with this group. At present, we do not believe that they produce long-term developmental changes in breastfed infants but this is not well documented.

The newer family of serotonin reuptake inhibitors (Prozac, Zoloft, Paxil) are widely popular, and have fewer side effects in adults. We do not know if they produce long-term changes in exposed infants. These drugs should be used with caution, and close observation by your physician.

Of this latter family, a number of side effects have been reported with Prozac (fluoxetine) (colic, nervousness,etc), so I no longer suggest its use. Newer reports with Zoloft (sertraline) suggest that little or none is absorbed by the infant, as we cannot find it in the infants blood. Paxil(paroxetine) may be another alternative, as its reported milk levels are exceedingly low. A great deal of interest in the new herbal product, St. John's Wort, has arisen. At present we have no data on its transfer to human milk, and I urge caution with this product.

In Conclusion

We are quite fortunate that most medications are safe to use while breastfeeding. We have strong data to support this. However, far too often, healthcare workers advise against using any medication whatsoever while breastfeeding because they are unfamiliar with using medications in breastfeeding mothers. Almost without exception, the product literature from all pharmaceutical firms recommends against breastfeeding. All of us know that this is unnecessarily cautious. Mothers should always question the necessity for using drugs while they are breastfeeding, but likewise, they should be strong in their conviction that breastfeeding is important to them and their infant, and be adamant that the doctor choose a medication that is both proper for the situation and safe for the baby.

Thomas W. Hale, R.Ph, Ph.D.
Associate Professor of Pediatrics
Division of Clinical Pharmacology and Toxicology
Texas Tech University School of Medicine
Amarillo, Texas

Dr. Hale is a pediatric clinical pharmacologist with many years of experience in pediatric medicine. He is the author of the best selling book, Medications and Mothers' Milk which is a compendium of almost 600 drugs and their use in lactating mothers. It is considered by many to be the most complete and up-to-date reference in this field.

It is available from: Pharmasoft Publishing
                             4606 Oregon
                             Amarillo, TX 79109
                             800-378-1317

                             Price 19.95 plus $3.00 shipping.

Sources for Breastfeeding Aids

The following companies manufacture or carry breast pumps which can be rented or purchased. They also carry breastfeeding aids such as breast shells, nipple shields, nursing pillows, nursing supplementers, slings, and other products for the nursing mother.

Ameda Egnell
765 Industrial Dr.
Cary IL 60013
(800) 323-8750

Bailey Medical Engineering (Nurture III)
2020 11th St.
Los Osos CA 93402
(805) 528-5781

Lact-Aid International, Inc. (nursing supplementers)
P. O. Box 1066
Athens TN 37371-1066

Medela, Inc.
P. O. Box 660
McHenry IL 60051
(800) 435-8316

Natural Choice
2073 Porter Lake Dr.
Sarasota FL 34240
(888)887-2229

Nifty Nurser (nursing pillows)
24307 Magic Mountain Pkwy.#118 Valencia CA 91355
(800) 296-9640

Over the Shoulder Baby Holder
P. O. Box 5191
San Clemente CA 92674
(800)637-9426

White River, Inc.
924 C. Calle Negocio
San Clemente CA 92673
(800) 824-6351

Mail Order Sources for Nursing Fashions
and Other Products for New Moms

Decent Exposure (Customer furnishes fabric for nursing fashions)
11 Treefern Place
Hampton VA 23666
(757) 825-0570

Diana Designs (T-shirts and other items with breastfeeding slogans for mom and baby)
160 River Forest
Fayetteville GA 30214

Medela, Inc. (Nursing bras and gowns)
P. O. Box 660
McHenry IL 60051
(800)435-8316

Motherwear, Inc. (Nursing fashions)
Box 114N1
Northampton MA 01061
(800)950-2500

NoMoreStretchMarks.com (An all-natural gel that will permanently fade away stretchmarks with an unconditional, 100% Money-Back Guarantee)
3422 Old Capital Trail Ste. 1215
Wilmington, DE 19808
Toll Free 877-NoMarks
http://www.NoMoreStretchMarks.com

Simply Delicious Nursingwear (Nursing fashions and Over the Shoulder Baby Holder)
P. O. Box 5191
San Clemente CA 92674
(800)637-9426

Mail-Order Bookstores that Carry Breastfeeding, Childbirth, and Parenting books

Birth and Life Bookstore
Division of Cascade Healthcare
141 Commercial St. NE
Salem OR 97301
(800)443-9942

Childbirth Graphics
Division of WRS , Inc.
P. O. Box 21207
Waco TX 76702
(800)299-3366

ICEA Bookcenter
P. O. Box 20048
Minneapolis MN 55420
(800)624-4934

La Leche League International
P. O. Box 4079
Schaumburg IL 60168
(847)519-0035

The Learning Curve of Weingart Design
4614 Prospect Ave. #421
Cleveland OH 44103
(800)795-9295

Good Books and Videos *

Breastfeeding: Biocultural Perspectives by Patricia Stuart-Macadam and Katherine Dettwyler

Breastfeeding: Pure and Simple by Gwen Gotsch,

Milk, Money & Madness: The Culture and Politics of Breastfeeding by Dia Michels and Naomi Baumslag

Mothering Multiples by Karen Gromada

Mothering Your Nursing Toddler by Norma Jane Bumgarner

Nighttime Parenting and *The Fussy Baby* by William Sears, MD

Womanly Art of Breastfeeding, by La Leche League International

A Healthier Baby by Breastfeeding by Linda Smith, IBCLC (video)

Breastfeeding Your Baby by Medela and LLLI (video)
* available at bookstores listed above

ABOUT THE AUTHOR

Pamela King Wiggins is an International Board Certified Lactation Consultant. Considered one of the "pioneers," she made the trek to Washington, D. C. to take the very first IBCLC examination in 1985. She currently teaches breastfeeding classes to expectant parents and presents in-services for nurses. She has previously worked for WIC, where she designed and initiated a lactation program in a Florida hospital. She has been counseling breastfeeding mothers for over two decades. She has a degree in liberal arts.

Pamela is a member of the International Lactation Consultant Association, the Tidewater Area Lactation Consultant Association and La Leche League International.

She is the author of *Why Should I Nurse My Baby?*, a popular guide used by hospitals and health departments all across the U. S. and Puerto Rico. It is available in English, Spanish, Creole and French.

Pamela is also the author of *Life in the Family Lane,* a collection of humorous and heart-warming essays taken from her popular magazine column of the same name.

The author, and her husband, Joe Nye Wiggins, have three children, Joe, Joanna and John, and one grandchild, Christopher John. They are also godparents to five healthy, breastfed boys, one of whom is featured on the cover of this book. The family lives on farm where they raise peanuts and pine trees.

INDEX

ORDER FORM

Breastfeeding: A Mother's Gift

Price: 9.95 + 2.00 shipping ($11.95) (Please call for bulk pricing.)

Also available:

Why Should I Nurse My Baby?
by Pamela K Wiggins, IBCLC

A 64 page, easy-to-read breastfeeding guide. Especially suitable for use in prenatal classes, WIC programs and hospital discharge packets.
Available in 4 languages. Bulk prices available.

Price: 4.95 + 1.55 shipping ($6.50) (Please call for bulk pricing.)

Specify: **English, Spanish, Creole or French.**

Send check or money order to: **L. A. Publishing Co.**
P. O. Box 773
Franklin VA 23851
or call: 1-800-397-5833

Name_____

Address _____

City & State _____Zip_____

Phone #_____
Please send me:

Breastfeeding: A Mother's Gift   ____   ($11.95 ea. enclosed)
Why Should I Nurse My Baby?   ____   ($6.50 ea. enclosed)

Or send Visa/MC number and expiration date
Virginia residents, add 4.5% sales tax